T0212016

Gynaecology in Primary Care

A PRACTICAL GUIDE

ANITA SHARMA

MBBS, MD, DRCOG, MFFP
General Practitioner
Oldham
Clinical Director, Vascular and Medicine Management
Oldham CCG

Forewords by

IAN WILKINSON
Chief Clinical Offi cer
NHS Oldham CCG

DENIS GIZZI
Managing Director
Oldham CCG

KATH WYNNE-JONES
Head of Programme Delivery and Business
Operations Oldham CCG

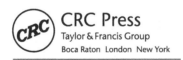

CRC Press
Taylor & Francis Group
Boca Raton London New York

CRC Press is an imprint of the
Taylor & Francis Group, an **informa** business

CRC Press
Taylor & Francis Group
6000 Broken Sound Parkway NW, Suite 300
Boca Raton, FL 33487-2742

© 2013 by Anita Sharma
CRC Press is an imprint of Taylor & Francis Group, an Informa business

No claim to original U.S. Government works

Printed on acid-free paper
Version Date: 20161202

International Standard Book Number-13: 978-1-84619-574-7 (Paperback)

This book contains information obtained from authentic and highly regarded sources. While all reasonable efforts have been made to publish reliable data and information, neither the author[s] nor the publisher can accept any legal responsibility or liability for any errors or omissions that may be made. The publishers wish to make clear that any views or opinions expressed in this book by individual editors, authors or contributors are personal to them and do not necessarily reflect the views/opinions of the publishers. The information or guidance contained in this book is intended for use by medical, scientific or health-care professionals and is provided strictly as a supplement to the medical or other professional's own judgement, their knowledge of the patient's medical history, relevant manufacturer's instructions and the appropriate best practice guidelines. Because of the rapid advances in medical science, any information or advice on dosages, procedures or diagnoses should be independently verified. The reader is strongly urged to consult the relevant national drug formulary and the drug companies' and device or material manufacturers' printed instructions, and their websites, before administering or utilizing any of the drugs, devices or materials mentioned in this book. This book does not indicate whether a particular treatment is appropriate or suitable for a particular individual. Ultimately it is the sole responsibility of the medical professional to make his or her own professional judgements, so as to advise and treat patients appropriately. The authors and publishers have also attempted to trace the copyright holders of all material reproduced in this publication and apologize to copyright holders if permission to publish in this form has not been obtained. If any copyright material has not been acknowledged please write and let us know so we may rectify in any future reprint.

Except as permitted under U.S. Copyright Law, no part of this book may be reprinted, reproduced, transmitted, or utilized in any form by any electronic, mechanical, or other means, now known or hereafter invented, including photocopying, microfilming, and recording, or in any information storage or retrieval system, without written permission from the publishers.

For permission to photocopy or use material electronically from this work, please access www.copyright.com (http://www.copyright.com/) or contact the Copyright Clearance Center, Inc. (CCC), 222 Rosewood Drive, Danvers, MA 01923, 978-750-8400. CCC is a not-for-profit organization that provides licenses and registration for a variety of users. For organizations that have been granted a photocopy license by the CCC, a separate system of payment has been arranged.

Trademark Notice: Product or corporate names may be trademarks or registered trademarks, and are used only for identification and explanation without intent to infringe.

Visit the Taylor & Francis Web site at
http://www.taylorandfrancis.com

and the CRC Press Web site at
http://www.crcpress.com

Contents

Foreword by Ian Wilkinson

Gynaecology in Primary Care comes at a time of great change in health service delivery. General practice is facing the challenges of developing clinical commissioning groups, providing ever greater range of primary care services, and implementing NICE guidelines while CCGs through their members will be under a legal duty to innovate. It is against this background that this textbook is particularly welcome.

Dr Sharma has produced an excellent text, supported by evidence, which acts as a guide to the management of gynaecological problems in primary care for not only clinicians in training, but for more experienced clinicians who look for straightforward and easily accessible advice to support their clinical management decisions. They need look no further than this textbook.

Clinical commissioning groups are required to improve the quality of primary care services and will need to address the problem of variation across their practice membership. Their promotion of best practice will be key to realising not only best health experience for individual patients but also best health outcomes for the population, while delivering within the current challenging financial environment. Dr Sharma's textbook will be a boon to developing organisations in delivering world-class services.

Dr Ian Wilkinson
Chief Clinical Officer
NHS Oldham CCG
February 2013

Foreword by Denis Gizzi

A further aspect concerning economies aiming for integrated service and clinical solutions is the way in which the constitutional rights of patients will be championed and delivered, via a system based on collaboration rather than merely competition. In addition to this is the requirement for new world commissioners (i.e. CCGs) to oversee and commission effective clinical contribution within all pathways of care, spanning total provider markets and care delivery systems.

Dr Anita Sharma has connected these clinical system management aspects with care pathway solutions. Optimal patient care requires many connected features to synchronise effectively; this book describes how this could be achieved by focusing attention on well-crafted, evidence-based clinical pathways. The public, in particular when they become patients or carers, justifiably expect high standards of support, care and advice. This book advances our thinking on how we connect clinical, system and patient level perspectives on optimal care management.

Denis Gizzi
Managing Director
Oldham CCG
February 2013

Foreword by Kath Wynne-Jones

Establishing integrated clinical pathways across providers should be at the heart of any CCG's strategy to ensure that high-quality, efficient services are commissioned on behalf of the population they serve. Effective management of patients within high-quality primary and community services will be the key to delivering the ambitions of many CCGs. However, it is crucial that such services are provided in line with the national evidence base. This is a responsibility which GPs must take on, both as primary care providers and as commissioners of the future.

From a provider perspective, this book aims to equip GPs with up-to-date knowledge of common gynaecological conditions, suggestions of best practice with regard to management and investigations to be undertaken within primary care, and guidelines for onward referral where appropriate and necessary. From a commissioning perspective, this book provides a valuable resource to CCGs, to inform their future pathways for gynaecological care.

Written by a highly regarded, experienced and practicing GP, who has taken on the role as Clinical Director on behalf of the CCG for this programme area, this book is a valuable asset for both practising GPs and developing CCGs to ensure that gynaecology services commission effectively, maximise the health of the population, improve the experience of the patient, and improve value for money.

Kath Wynne-Jones BSc, MPhil
Head of Programme Delivery and Business Operations
Oldham CCG
February 2013

Preface

National Institute for Health and Clinical Excellence (NICE) quality standards are being developed to make it clear to service providers what quality care means. Quality standards for some clinical areas have already been published and some will be published over the next five years, but gynaecological care has thus far been ignored. The quality standards are a set of specific, concise statements that are based on best available evidence and which act as markers of high-quality cost-effective patient care.

The clinical commissioning world is a brave new world, which commissioners will take into account when planning and delivering services as part of a general duty to secure continuous improvement in quality and to provide better care for our patients, in the right place and at the right time. I welcome these changes and as a GP would like to see women's health high on the agenda – not only to maintain but also to improve the standards of women's healthcare.

Inadequate primary care management, and an early referral to secondary care, is bound to raise concerns from secondary care colleagues that patients are not receiving the appropriate treatment when in primary care. There may be complaints of poor-quality referral letters with no examination findings, or a lack of routine investigations. This highlights a need for improved education in the primary care setting. It is acknowledged that primary care needs to have a broader knowledge of many common gynaecological problems. This book gives you, the reader, best practices for management of common gynaecological conditions, alongside summaries of new research, pulling out key points and recommending actions you might consider taking before referring a patient.

For a busy GP there are simply not enough hours in a day to read all the research that is available. I have added to each chapter relevant research and RCOG guidelines that will mean you won't have to spend unnecessary hours on the internet.

With the emergence of clinical commissioning groups, commissioners should consider establishing specialist community services to reduce lengthy waiting lists, increasing choice for women while reducing economic costs. By developing a patient pathway as per nationally agreed guidelines, the management of conditions like abnormal uterine bleeding, menopause, pessary change for prolapse and incontinence can be easily provided in the primary care setting, led by a GP with a special interest in gynaecology. This book is written to deliver the main aim of the RCP report, which is to ensure the best care for our female patients in a setting of their choice, and to develop streamlined one-stop services in primary care so that women do not have to take time off from work and family commitments.

I regard this book as the start of an evolutionary process and the first of many editions. What better time for me as a female GP to share my innovative ideas and provide a practical guide to gynaecology in primary care than when The Royal College of General Practitioners has a female president. I want to make sure that women's healthcare does not become a casualty of the new NHS by encouraging all readers to become actively involved in clinical commissioning groups' decisions as to which services should take a priority in their area. This book offers plenty of ideas.

Gynaecology in Primary Care: a practical guide is intended primarily for general practitioners but will be of value to other healthcare professionals and medical students. If you gain greater gynaecological knowledge, develop a one-stop pathway in your area and reduce the number of referrals to secondary care, the book will have served its purpose well.

Anita Sharma
February 2013

About the author

Anita Sharma MBBS, MD, DRCOG, MFFP has been a general practitioner in Oldham for more than 24 years and loves every second of working as a GP.

She is an undergraduate trainer attached to the University of Manchester and a trainer in family planning. She is the GP editor for the *British Journal of Medical Practitioners*. She writes regularly in various GP magazines on clinical and practice developmental issues.

Anita has served as a Local Medical Committee locality member for the last 7 years and is a GP appraiser for Oldham Primary Care Trust. She is also the chairperson of BMA Rochdale Division where she organises various educational and social activities.

With the help and support of her patient participation group, she organises various fundraising activities and raises money for Cancer Research. She has written three books, all aimed towards the primary care physician: *COPD in Primary Care* (Radcliffe Publishing, 2010), *Peripheral Vascular Disease in Primary Care* (Radcliffe Publishing, 2011), and *Maximising Quality and Outcomes Framework Quality Points* (Radcliffe Publishing, 2011). She donates her royalties raised by *COPD in Primary Care* to the 'Breathe Easy' group.

She was a GP member of the NICE lower limb peripheral arterial disease guideline development group. She contributed on clinical audit tool and secondary prevention from a GP perspective.

Anita is also the clinical director in vascular and medicine management of the Oldham Clinical Commissioning Group (CCG). She is actively involved in the setting up of one-stop gynaecological and early pregnancy assessment services in Oldham.

Acknowledgements

Every piece of writing takes time – the time that could have been spent with my husband and children.

My heartfelt gratitude goes to my husband, Ravi, a consultant physician, for his continued support and doing my household duties while I battled with my computer.

Above all, I would like to thank my son Neel and daughter Ravnita.

I am indebted to Dr Grace Edozien for her contribution towards current approaches to managing dysfunctional uterine bleeding. She describes a clear pathway for patients presenting in primary care with postmenopausal and postcoital bleeding.

The management of cancer is complex. Early diagnosis and multidisciplinary specialist management plays a key role. I thank Dr Theofanis Manias and Gill Barnes for explaining how the management needs to be planned on an individualised basis, taking into account the extent of disease at presentations as per NICE guidelines.

The author would like to thank Dr Catherine Mammen for the expert guidance she has offered in relation to understanding pelvic ultrasound scan.

General practice is the first point of contact for many women seeking advice on infertility. I am grateful indeed to Dr Shalini Gadiyar for explaining what general advice and specific treatments are available, and if the couple is referred to the hospital, what further tests they might anticipate.

Dr Uma Marthi explains the new criteria for defining polycystic ovary syndrome. I am thankful to her for making it easy for the reader to understand how to diagnose and treat one of the most common endocrine disorders affecting women during their reproductive years.

Vaginal discharge is a common presenting problem in general practice and I am particularly grateful to Dr Sarup Tayal for his contribution on its assessment and management in primary care. He provides an excellent guide for primary care physicians on which patients should be referred.

I would like to record my sincere thanks to Michael Dearden and the newly commissioned pessary service in Oldham which offers a vision of truly 21st century healthcare for women closer to home.

I particularly wish to thank Heather Mallison and Helen Taylor of Oldham

Primary Care Trust for their help in the preparation of the illustrations, graphs and tables.

My thanks also go to the patients who have given consent for the use of ultrasound scan photographs in this book.

Finally, I thank Camille Lowe and Jamie Etherington for their continuing support and help with the preparation of the manuscript.

As will become apparent to all who read this book, I have long been driven by high-quality personal care, continuity of care and a commitment to patients which makes being a GP with a Special Interest in Gynaecology a profession rather than just a job. I sincerely hope that you, the readers, agree that this has been time well spent.

Anita Sharma
GPwSI in Gynaecology

Dysmenorrhoea

DEFINITION

Dysmenorrhoea is defined as painful menstruation that interferes with a woman's physical, emotional and social quality of life.[1] The term dysmenorrhoea is derived from the Greek words *dys* meaning difficult/painful, *meno*, meaning month and *rrhea*, meaning flow.

Dysmenorrhoea is one of the most common gynaecological problems in young women who present to their general practitioner. Menstrual pain is often described as lower abdominal cramp-like pain, sharp/aching pain that comes and goes, or sometimes back pain during the period. Some pain during periods is normal but excessive pain must not be ignored. Premenstrual symptoms are often present including nausea and vomiting.

It is classified as either primary (spasmodic) or secondary (congestive) dysmenorrhoea.

Primary dysmenorrhoea is defined as recurrent, cramp-like pain occurring during menstruation in the absence of any pelvic pathology. It usually begins in adolescence. Current evidence suggests that primary dysmenorrhoea is due to prostaglandin F2 alpha (PGF2 alpha), a potent myometrial stimulant and vasoconstrictor present in the secretory endometrium.[2] This causes an increased myometrial activity resulting in uterine ischemia and pain. The uterine contractions can last many minutes and may produce uterine pressures greater than 60 mmHg. Elevated levels of prostaglandin were found in the endometrial fluid of women with dysmenorrhoea and the level found correlated with the degree of pain.[3]

Pathophysiology of primary dysmenorrhoea:

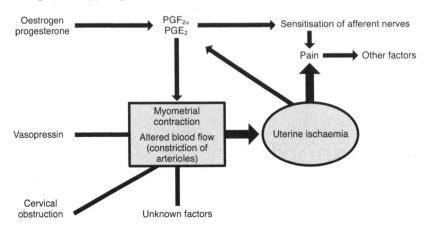

FIGURE 1.1 Pathophysiology of primary dysmenorrhoea
Source: Primary Dysmenorrhoea Consensus Guideline
www.sogc.org/guidelines/public/169E-CPG-December2005.pdf

Secondary dysmenorrhoea is defined as menstrual pain resulting from gynaecological pathology, e.g. fibroids, endometriosis or pelvic inflammatory disease.

Prevalence

Dysmenorrhoea is one of the most common gynaecological problems in young women presenting to clinicians.[4]

Its prevalence is estimated at 25% in women of all age groups. It is most common in adolescents. Ninety per cent of female adolescents tend to suffer with dysmenorrhoea.[5] Primary dysmenorrhoea affects up to 50% of postpubertal women.[6] Secondary dysmenorrhoea is most common in women aged 30–45 years. Dysmenorrhoea severe enough to cause absence from work occurs in less than 5% of women.[7]

Risk factors

The following risk factors have been associated with severe episodes of dysmenorrhoea:[8]
- smoking
- early menarche
- heavy menstrual bleed
- prolonged menstrual bleed

- strong family history
- obesity
- age (symptoms are more pronounced in adolescents than in older women)[7]
- lower socioeconomic groups[4]
- frequent lifestyle changes, less social support and stressful relationships.[9]

Obesity and excess alcohol consumption were found to be associated with dysmenorrhoea in some (but not all) studies.[10,11] Physical activity is not thought to be associated with dysmenorrhoea.[8] There is some evidence that parous women have less severe dysmenorrhoea.[2,10]

Primary care management

The optimal management depends on distinguishing between primary and secondary dysmenorrhoea. Although it is not life threatening, it can be debilitating and it is essential that the underlying pathology is identified and treated specifically.

Women suffering from primary dysmenorrhoea do not usually seek medical help and do not make use of available prescription medications. A detailed gynaecological history can easily distinguish between primary and secondary dysmenorrhoea.

History
Menstrual history
Enquire as to the age of menarche, length and duration of bleeding and whether associated with blood clots.

Pain
Enquire about the type, duration, radiation of pain, association with any other symptoms (bladder/bowel), severity and the degree of disability. Ask about all therapies used in the past for pain relief including over-the-counter preparations.

Sexual history
It is important to ask about sexual history, past history of sexually transmitted infections (STIs), vaginal discharge and dyspareunia. Enquire about contraception. Many adolescents use dysmenorrhoea as a pretext to seek contraception.

Family history:
Enquire about any family history of endometriosis. A family history of endometriosis may be an indicator for referral.

Andersch and Milsom categorised dysmenorrhoea in grades 0–3:[11]

Grade 0   No pain, no effect on activity.
Grade 1   Mild pain, activity seldom affected, analgesics seldom needed.
Grade 2   Moderate pain, activity affected, analgesics required, seldom absent from school or work.
Grade 3   Severe pain, activity inhibited, analgesics poorly effective. Vegetative symptoms present.

TABLE 1.1 How to differentiate between primary and secondary dysmenorrhoea

HISTORY	PRIMARY	SECONDARY
Age	16–25 years	30–45 years
Onset	Since menarche	Later than menarche
Pain	Commences with the start of period	Noncyclical and cyclical episodes
Duration	8–72 hours during menses	Variable number of days, prior to +/– throughout the cycle
Nature of pain	Cramps like pain	Chronic pelvic pain associated with heavy bleeds/dyspareunia and possible bowel and urological symptoms
Co-morbidity	No associated gynaecological, gastrointestinal or urological problems	Associated with various gynae symptoms. May present with GI or urological symptoms
Benefit with NSAIDs or COC	Yes	No/slight benefit
Clinical examination	Normal	Normal or tender uterus/ adnexae/ enlarged uterus/adnexae
Pelvic ultrasound scan	Normal	Normal/fibroid/ adenomyosis ovarian cyst/mass

Source: www.prescriber.co.uk Reproduced with the permission of Wiley.

Investigations

Essential investigations in primary care are ultrasound examination, high vaginal, gonococcal and chlamydial swabs. There is no evidence for the routine use of ultrasound scanning in all patients presenting with dysmenorrhoea. Ultrasound is indicated in:

- women with an abnormality on pelvic examination – tender or enlarged uterus or an adnexal mass

- women for whom a pelvic examination is impossible or unsatisfactory
- women refractory to first-line therapy.

Differential diagnosis of secondary dysmenorrhoea:
- endometriosis
- fibroids
- pelvic inflammatory disease
- ovarian cysts
- endometrial polyps
- cervical stenosis
- imperforate hymen or congenital Müllerian anomalies.

Treatment
Conservative
- Reassure the patient that this is not a disease but a well-recognised condition that tends to improve with time. In 19-year-olds, after 5 years, prevalence falls from 72% to 67%, and the percentage experiencing limitation in daily activity decreases from 51% to 34%. In addition, dysmenorrhoea may improve after childbirth.[10,13]
- Engagement in decision making about the management has a positive benefit and patients obtain more relief.[14]
- Heat: applying heat to the lower abdomen with a heating pad or hot water bottle can reduce the pain and can be applied as soon as the pain starts, as often as needed. A temperature of 104 degrees Fahrenheit or 40 degrees Celsius is recommended.
- Exercise: may improve dysmenorrhoea, but controlled trials have been small and of poor quality and the results of trials have been mixed.[15] Exercise increases general health, both physically and psychologically, and must therefore be recommended.
- Smoking cessation, alcohol intake reduction, weight loss and stress reduction all have positive health benefits and must be recommended to patients. It is not known whether modifying these factors decreases symptoms.[16]
- Dietary supplements: have not shown to be beneficial[17] but can have a placebo effect.[18]
- Complementary therapy like yoga: there is some evidence that yoga may be beneficial in relieving pain but further studies are needed. Further information about complementary and alternative medicine is available at: http://nccam.nih.gov/.
- High frequency transcutaneous electric nerve stimulation (TENS): this can be a suitable alternative in women who do not wish to take medication, although not proved to be effective.[19]

- Acupuncture or behavioural therapy may be beneficial in some cases.[16]

Drug therapy

- Simple analgesia: paracetamol or combination of paracetamol and codeine in small doses is effective in most women. If prescribing opioids, the risk of addiction must be carefully considered.
- Non-steroidal anti-inflammatory drugs (NSAIDs): these work by inhibiting prostaglandin synthesis and reducing myometrial contractions. They are most effective if started as soon as bleeding or other menstrual symptoms begin and then taken on a regular basis for 2–3 days. Although there is little difference in efficacy between different

TABLE 1.2 At a glance management

VALUE OF TREATMENT	TYPE OF TREATMENT	LEVEL OF SUPPORTING EVIDENCE*
Beneficial	NSAIDs (other than aspirin)	A
Likely to be beneficial	Combined oral contraceptives	B, C
	Progestogens, e.g. LNG-IUS	B, C
	Acupressure	C
	Aspirin, paracetamol and compound analgesics	B, C
	TENS (high-frequency stimulation only; effects of low-frequency stimulation remain unclear)	B
	Tropical heat (about 39 degrees C)	C
Unknown effectiveness	Fish oil	C
	Herbal remedies other than toki-shakuyaku-san	C
	Magnesium	C
	Magnets	C
	Surgical interruption of pelvic nerve pathways	C
	Vitamin B12	C
Unlikely to be beneficial	Spinal manipulation	C

*Classification of evidence (US Agency for Health Care Research and Quality):

A: requires at least 1 randomised controlled trial as part of a body of literature of overall good quality and consistency addressing the specific recommendation (evidence levels Ia, Ib).

B: requires the availability of well-controlled clinical studies but no randomised clinical trials on the topic of recommendations (evidence levels IIa, IIb, III).

C: requires evidence obtained from expert committee reports or opinions and/or clinical experiences of respected authorities; indicates an absence of directly applicable clinical studies of good quality (evidence level IV).

Source: Evidence-based treatment options for primary dysmenorrhoea, 5 June 2009: www. prescriber.co.uk

NSAIDs, a small randomised double-blind placebo-controlled trial concluded that diclofenac restored exercise performance as assessed by aerobic capacity.[20]

- Combined oral contraceptive pill (COC): this acts by inhibiting ovulation, inducing endometrial thinning and lowering the level of uterine prostaglandin. This results in not only lighter but also less painful periods. The COC – even the cyclical low-dose monophasic pill – decreases analgesic use and disability in patients with primary dysmenorrhoea.[21] The 'tricycling regime' – running three packets together without the 7-day break – reduces frequency of bleeds further. The combined contraceptive pill is also effective in reducing pain due to endometriomata.[22] A combination of NSAIDs and COCs may be a reasonable option if case of inadequate benefit with a single medication.[16]

- Progesterone-only contraceptive pill (POP): Cerazette (desogestrel) has been shown to relieve dysmenorrhoea in one observational study.[23] It can be used in women who experience oestrogenic side effects. Depot medroxyprogesterone acetate (Depo-Provera) also suppresses ovulation and improves dysmenorrhoea.

- The levonorgestrel-releasing intrauterine system (Mirena) can be beneficial in reducing menstrual loss and pain but is not licensed as a treatment for dysmenorrhoea.

- Glyceryl trinitrite (GTN) patches, not used routinely, were shown to relieve dysmenorrhoea in a randomised controlled trial (RCT).[24]

Treatment options that may be considered by a gynaecologist
- COCP
- Depo Provera
- Gonadotrophin-releasing analogues
- Laparoscopy and ablation of endometriosis/adhesiolysis/ (resection of endometriotic tissue, neurectomy in severe cases)
- Hysterectomy and/or bilateral salpingo-oophorectomy

FIGURE 1.2 Treatment options that may be considered by a gynaecologist
Source: Modern management of dysmenorrhoea. Thomas B, Magos A. *Trends in Urology Gynaecology and Sexual Health*. Sep/Oct 2009; **15**(5): 25–9. www.tugsh.com

Surgical

- Thermal ablation of endometriosis if the cause is endometriosis.
- Presacral neurectomy (PSN) and uterine nerve ablation (UNA) reserved for severe cases.[25]

Referral to secondary care

- Suspicion of endometriosis (history of dyspareunia, dysmenorrhoea, painful defecation, pelvic pain), pelvic inflammatory disease (PID) or pelvic adhesions with a view to laparoscopy.
- Abnormal ultrasound report – fibroid, adenomyosis, ovarian cyst, tubo-ovarian mass.
- Patients with long-standing severe symptoms and no significant improvement with non steroidal inflammatory drugs (NSAIDs) and or combined oral contraceptives (COCs).

KEY POINTS

- The majority of patients with dysmenorrhoea have no underlying pathology and can be managed by a GP.
- Painful periods become less common as women experience ageing.
- Providing explanation and reassurance is all that is needed in most cases.
- Most patients respond to simple analgesia, NSAIDs and COCs.

Useful websites

For GPs

The American College of Obstetricians and Gynaecologists: www.nlm.nih.gov/medlineplus/ency/article/003150.htm

Primary dysmenorrhoea consensus guideline: www.acog.org/For_Patients www.sogc.org/jogc/...CPD_abstract-jogc/.../CPD-abstract-JOGC-dec-05.pdf

References

1 Proctor ML, Farquhar CM. Dysmenorrhoea. *Clin Evid.* Jun 2006; (15): 2429–48.
2 Willman EA, Collins WP, Clayton SG. Studies in the involvement of prostaglandins in uterine symptomatology and pathology. *Br J Obstet Gynaecol.* 1976; **83**(5): 337–41.
3 Eden JA. Dysmenorrhoea and premenstrual syndrome. In: Hacker NF, Moore JG, editors. *Essentials of Obstetrics and Gynecology.* 3rd ed. Philadelphia, PA: WB Saunders; 1998. pp. 386–92.

4 Jamieson DJ, Steege JF. The prevalence of dysmenorrhea, dyspareunia, pelvic pain and irritable bowel syndrome in primary care practices. *Obstet Gynecol.* Jan 1996; **87**(1): 55–8.

5 Durain D. Primary dysmenorrhea assessment and management update. *J Midwifery Women's Health.* Nov–Dec 2004; **49**(6): 520–8.

6 Dawood MY. Nonsteroidal anti-inflammatory drugs and changing attitudes toward dysmenorrhoea. *Am J Med.* 20 May 1988; **84**(5A): 23–9.

7 Weissman AM, Hartz AY, Hansen MD, *et al.* The natural history of primary dysmenorrhoea: a longitudinal study. *BJOG.* Apr 2004; **111**(4): 345–52.

8 Harlow SD, Park M. A longitudinal study of risk factors for the occurrence, duration and severity of menstrual cramps in a cohort of college women. *Br J Obstet Gynaecol.* Nov 1996; **103**(11): 1134–42.

9 Alonso C, Coe CL. Disruptions of social relationship accentuate the association between emotional distress and menstrual pain in young women. *Health Psychol.* 2001; **20**(6): 411–6.

10 Sundell G, Milsom I, Andersch B. Factors influencing the prevalence and severity of dysmenorrhoea in young women. *Br J Obstet Gynaecol.* Jul 1990; **97**(7): 588–94.

11 Andersch B, Milsom I. An epidemiologic study of young women with dysmenorrhea. *Am J Obstet Gynecol.* Nov 15, 1982; **144**(6): 655–60.

12 Dysmenorrhoea Monograph: www.wholehealthmedia.com/Dysmenorrhea%20 PDF.pdf

13 Weissman AM, Hartz AJ, Hansen MD, *et al.* The natural history of primary dysmenorrhoea: a longitudinal study. *Br J Obstet Gynaecol.* 2004; **111**: 345–52.

14 Ballagh SA, Heyl A. Communicating with women about menstrual cycle symptoms. *J Reprod Med.* 2008; **53**(11): 837–46.

15 Daley AJ. Exercise and primary dysmenorrhoea: a comprehensive and critical review of the literature. *Sports Med.* 2008; **38**(8): 659–70.

16 Wills H, Demetriou C, May K, Kennedy S, *et al. NHS Evidence – Women's Health Dysmenorrhoea. Annual Evidence Update March 2010.* Oxford: Nuffield Department of Obstetrics and Gynaecology, University of Oxford; 2010. Available at: arms.evidence.nhs.uk/resources/hub/350909/attachment

17 Proctor ML, Murphy PA. Herbal and dietary therapies for primary and secondary dysmenorrhoea. *Cochrane Database Syst Rev.* 2001; 3(CD002124).

18 Cheng JF, Lu ZY, Su YC, *et al.* A traditional Chinese herbal medicine used to treat dysmenorrhoea among Taiwanese women. *J Clin Nurs.* 2008; **17**(19): 2588–95.

19 Proctor M, Smith CA, Farquhar CM, *et al.* Transcutaneous electric nerve stimulation and acupuncture for primary dysmenorrhoea. *Cochrane Database Syst Rev.* 2002; 1(CD002123).

20 Chantler I, Mitchell D, Fuller A. Diclofenac potassium attenuates dysmenorrhoea and restores exercise performance in women with primary dysmenorrhoea. *J Pain.* 2009; **10**(2): 191–200.

21 MacDonald M. After 3 months, low dose oral contraceptives reduced pain in adolescent girls with moderate to severe dysmenorrhoea. *Evid Based Nurs.* 2006; **9**(1): 16.

22 Harada T, Momoeda M, Taketani Y, *et al.* Low dose oral contraceptive pill for dysmenorrhoea associated with endometriosis: a placebo-controlled, double-blind, randomised trial. *Fertil Steril.* 2008; **90**(5): 1583–8.

23 Ahrendt HJ, Karcht U, PichI T, *et al.* The effects of an oestrogen-free, desogestrel-containing oral contraceptive in women with cyclical symptoms: results from two studies on oestrogen-related symptoms and dysmenorrhoea. *Eur J Contracept Reprod Health Care.* 2007; **12**(4): 354–61.

24 Modares M, Rahnama P. Side effects of glyceryl trinitrate ointment for primary dysmenorrhoea: a randomised clinical trial. *Tehran Univ Med.* 2008; **65**(10): 61–6.

25 Lee TT, Yang LC. Pelvic denervation procedures: a current reappraisal. *Int J Gynaecol Obstet.* 2008; **101**(3): 304–8.

2

Premenstrual syndrome

DEFINITION

Premenstrual syndrome (PMS) is a condition characterised by somatic, behavioural, emotional and psychological symptoms during the luteal phase of the menstrual cycle. The symptoms become more intense in the 2–3 days prior to the period and usually resolve with the onset of menstruation. The symptoms can become so severe that they can impair functioning levels at work or school. The symptoms of PMS are related to ovulation.

Prevalence

The true prevalence rate is not known because of the great variation in the criteria for diagnosis. Around 20%–30% of menstruating women are believed to suffer from PMS. A patient who has had a hysterectomy can suffer from PMS if one ovary is remaining. About 3%–8% of women suffer from a severe condition called premenstrual dysphoric disorder (PMDD). Women with PMDD experience more severe symptoms.[1]

Aetiology

The precise aetiology of PMS is unknown. Cyclical ovarian activity and the effect of oestradiol and progesterone on the neurotransmitters serotonin and gamma amino butyric acid (GABA) appear to be the key factors. Genetic predisposition is also thought to be a contributory factor.

Diagnosis

The International Society for Premenstrual Disorders (ISPMD) has defined precise criteria for diagnosing premenstrual disorder. Correct diagnosis is essential for management. In an ovulating woman, the symptoms occur during the second half of the cycle and disappear by the end of menstruation. More than 150 symptoms have been reported to be associated with premenstrual syndrome (PMS). They can be physical, psychological or behavioural symptoms. Diagnosis depends not on the type or severity of the symptoms but on their timing.

Criteria of diagnosis:[2]

- symptoms precipitated by ovulation
- symptoms occurring in the second half of the cycle
- symptoms disappearing by the end of menstruation
- any number of symptoms can be present, ranging in severity
- mainly physical and psychological symptoms
- symptoms causing a lot of impairment of social, occupational and academic activities.[3]

Symptoms

Symptoms can be physical, psychological or behavioural.[2] A small percentage of women with severe psychological symptoms will also fulfil the American Psychiatric Association (APA) criteria for premenstrual dysphoric disorder.[4]

Physical symptoms:[3]

- headaches
- breast tenderness
- change of appetite
- constipation/diarrhoea
- puffiness of face, abdomen or fingers
- exacerbation of migraine, rhinitis, asthma or urticaria
- weight gain
- painful joints
- muscle aches/pains.

Psychological and behavioural symptoms:[3]

- sleep disorders
- aggression
- irritability
- mood swings/depression
- tearfulness
- food cravings
- difficulty concentrating
- tiredness
- confusion

- social withdrawal
- altered interest in sex.

TABLE 2.1 Types of premenstrual syndrome: based on symptoms

TYPE	DEFINITION
Mild	Does not interfere with personal/social or working life
Moderate	Interferes with personal/social and working life but woman is still able to function and interact, although may be suboptimal
Severe	Woman is unable to interact socially/professionally; withdrawn and treatment-resistant

Primary care management

It is important to make a correct diagnosis as this is a prerequisite for successful management. The woman should be asked to record her symptoms over two cycles as recommended in the Royal College of Obstetricians and Gynaecologists guidelines.[5] The Royal College recommends the daily recording of severity of symptoms. An internet-based tool may be used (www.symptometrics.com). It is worth remembering that cycle lengths vary. The average cycle is 28 days. In shorter cycles, the follicular phase may be only a few days long and symptoms are present for a greater proportion of time.

History

A proper history will enable you to decide whether it is mild, moderate or severe PMS. Enquire about the following.
- A detailed menstrual history: length, duration, regularity of the cycle, any associated pain and the date of the last menstrual period (LMP).
- History of premenstrual symptoms: timing of symptoms, what symptoms, severity of symptoms, absence or presence of symptoms after periods.
- Any medication taken: over the counter (OTC) or prescribed and any benefit received?
- Any effect on work, social activities, family, partner or hobbies? Time off from school or work?
- Contraceptive history: current contraception, e.g. combined or progesterone contraceptive pill.
- Any associated gynaecological history, e.g. endometriosis, dyspareunia, heavy menstrual bleeding?
- History of hormone replacement therapy (HRT).
- Any suicidal thoughts?

Differential diagnosis

- Thyroid disorders: exclude by doing thyroid function tests (TFTs).
- Anxiety and depression: exclude by doing hospital anxiety and depression scale score (HADS) or patient health questionnaire (PHQ-9) score.

Pelvic examination

A pelvic examination is not needed unless clinically indicated, especially if there is a history of heavy menstrual bleeding.

Management

Treatment regimes may take up to 3 months to make a difference in symptoms. More aggressive treatment is needed sooner rather than later at the severe end of the spectrum.

- A sympathetic ear and reassurance to the patient that PMS affects many women and that she is not 'going mad', is all that is needed most of the time.
- Education about PMS can be therapeutic for some women.
- Simple health promotion advice: regular aerobic exercise at least 20–30 minutes three times a week, healthy eating, reducing smoking/alcohol intake, relaxation and stress avoidance. Regular exercise has been shown to alleviate premenstrual symptoms. This is due to endorphin release and weight control.[17]
- A referral to a health trainer, smoking cessation counsellor or a clinical psychologist for CBT if clinically indicated. Cognitive behavioural therapy has been shown to help[18] but the evidence of reflexology and acupuncture is sparse.
- Supplements: calcium 1 g/day plus vitamin D 10 μg/day, magnesium oxide (250 mg/day), vitamin B_6 supplements (maximum 50 mg/day). The only herbal supplement shown to be effective in a small placebo-controlled trial is the fruit extract of *Vitex agnus-castus*.[6] Placebo-controlled studies show that calcium, vitamin B_6 and exercise may be superior to placebo. A programme of 10 cognitive behavioural therapy sessions (CBTs) has been found to be more effective when compared with fluoxetine given for 6 months.[7]
- Anxiolytics: buspirone 10–60 mg/day OR alprazolam 0.25 mg–4.0 mg twice or three times a day have been shown to be superior to placebo in placebo-controlled studies.[8] A systematic review found them ineffective.[9] *My personal view is that these drugs should not be initiated in primary care.*
- Diuretics: aldosterone antagonist spironolactone given only in luteal phase 100 mg/day can reduce the fluid retention and bloated

feeling of the lower abdomen.[10] *It is not licensed for this indication; remember to let the patient know and document in the notes.* The main contraindications are hyperkalaemia and anuria (*check urea and electrolytes before initiating and during treatment*).

- Psychotropic drugs: selective serotonin reuptake inhibitors (SSRIs) – fluoxetine, citalopram, sertraline and paroxetine – OR serotonin and noradrenaline reuptake inhibitors (SNRIs) – venlafaxine given in a daily dose or in the luteal phase (14 days before menses) – have been found to be effective in some placebo-controlled trials in treating mood disorders.[11] *SSRIs are not licensed in the United Kingdom for the management of premenstrual dysphoric disorder. Again document clearly in the notes if a prescription is issued for this indication. Inform the patient about the common side effect of decreased libido with continuous use.*

- Combined oral contraceptive pills (COCs): COCs work by suppressing ovulation. The majority of COCs contain ethinylestradiol as the oestrogen component; mestranol and estradiol valerate are also available. The ethinylestradiol content ranges from 20 to 35 µg. Ideally a preparation with a lower oestrogenic and progestogenic component should be chosen. COCs not only give a good cycle control, but also reduce dysmenorrhoea and menorrhagia symptoms. A 20 µg pill does have a higher rate of break-through bleeding. A newer oral contraceptive pill that contains 20 µg of ethinylestradiol and drospirenone with antiandrogenic and weak diuretic properties (Yasmin) suppresses ovulation and treats symptoms effectively according to two randomised controlled trials.[12,13] *Remember Yasmin is the most expensive COC (£14.70 for a three-cycle pack) and you may have to convince your medicine management team if your patient needs this for a longer period.*

- Progestogens: norethisterone, levonorgestrel and medroxyprogesterone acetate given in the luteal phase are the only agents licensed for managing premenstrual syndrome in the United Kingdom. A systematic review showed they are ineffective and often cause worsening of symptoms.[14] These drugs are only beneficial for endometrial protection during treatment with oestrogens to suppress ovulation.

- Danazol: danazol inhibits pituitary gonadotrophins. It combines androgenic activity with antioestrogenic and antiprogestogenic activity. A randomised placebo-controlled crossover trial found danazol of considerable benefit over placebo in the treatment of patients with premenstrual syndrome.[15]

- Gonadotropin-releasing hormone analogue (GnRH):

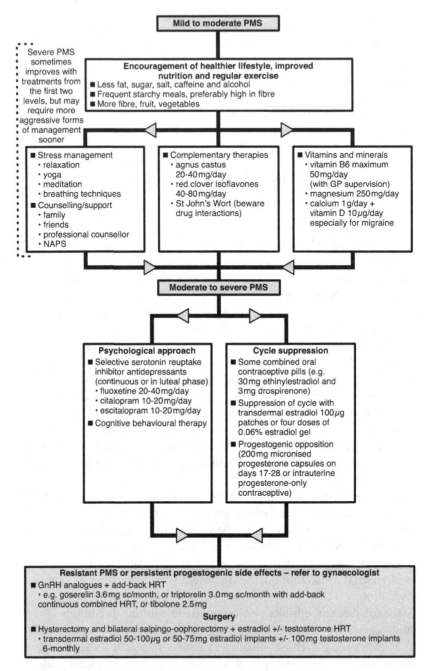

FIGURE 2.1 Treatment guidelines for premenstrual syndrome

Source: National Association for Premenstrual Syndrome (NAPS): www.guidelines.co.uk

Zoladex (goserelin). GnRH suppresses ovarian steroid production resulting in a medical menopause. Several randomised controlled trials have shown that GnRH agonists are effective in relieving symptoms of premenstrual disorders.[16]

- Surgery: A hysterectomy will eliminate periods but not premenstrual symptoms because ovarian function is conserved. Bilateral oophorectomy is indicated in exceptional circumstances, in women with severe debilitating symptoms. These women will need oestrogens until the age of natural menopause. A woman who is undergoing a hysterectomy for another gynaecological condition may consider having an oophorectomy to avoid ongoing premenstrual symptoms.

KEY POINTS

- Precise diagnosis is the key to successful treatment in most patients.
- There is no objective diagnostic test and diagnosis depends on the woman recording symptoms over two cycles as recommended in RCOG guidelines.
- A majority of women will need reassurance, support and advice about good nutrition, exercise and stress reduction. All this can easily be provided by a primary care physician.
- Regular exercise has been shown to alleviate premenstrual symptoms. This is due to endorphin release and weight control.[17]
- Cognitive behavioural therapy has been shown to help.[18]
- Complementary and over-the-counter preparations may be helpful but it is important to remember that beneficial evidence for their use is limited.
- SSRIs have been shown to be far superior to placebo in helping symptoms of PMS. They are most effective if taken continuously. *SSRIs are not licensed in the United Kingdom for the management of premenstrual dysphoric disorder.*
- A woman with severe debilitating symptoms and no symptom-free days may have underlying mental or psychological problems. Referral to a psychiatrist or counsellor may be needed in such cases.

Useful websites

For patients – helplines

Health information on premenstrual syndrome from the US National Library of Medicine: Medline Plus, www.nlm.nih.gov/medlineplus/premenstrualsyndrome.html

National Association for Premenstrual Syndrome: www.pms.org.uk

Patient information leaflet on managing premenstrual syndrome: www.rcog.org.uk/managing-premenstrual-syndrome-pms-information-you

Useful websites
For GPs
Evidence based, practice-informed care maps for the management of PMS: Map of Medicine, http://eng.mapofmedicine.com/evidence/map/menstrual_cycle_irregularities_and_post_menopausal_bleeding_pmb_7.html

Overview of premenstrual dysphoric disorder: Medscape, http://emedicine.medscape.com/article/293257-overview

Management of premenstrual syndrome: Royal College of Obstetricians and Gynaecologists (2007), www.rcog.org.uk/files/rcog-corp/uploaded-files/GT48ManagementPremensturalSyndrome.pdf

References

1 Emedicinehealth. Premenstrual syndrome (PMS): definition, causes and treatment. Available at: www.emedicinehealth.com/premenstrual_syndrome_pms/article_em.htm (accessed 6 December 2012).

2 O'Brien PM, Backstrom T, Brown C, *et al.* Towards a consensus on diagnostic criteria, measurement and trial design of the premenstrual disorders: the ISPMD Montreal consensus. *Arch Womens Ment Health.* 2011; **14**(1): 13–21.

3 Halbreich U, Borenstein J, Pearlstein T, *et al.* The prevalence, impairment, impact and burden of premenstrual dysphoric disorder (PMS/PMDD). *Psychoneuroendocrinology.* 2003; **28**(3): 1–23.

4 Dennerstein L, Lehert P, Keung LS, *et al.* A population-based survey of Asian women's experience of premenstrual symptoms. *Menopause Int.* 2010; **16**(4): 139–45.

5 Royal College of Obstetricians and Gynaecologists (RCOG). Premenstrual syndrome. Green-top guideline 48. RCOG Press; 2007. Available at: www.rcog.org.uk/files/rcog-corp/uploaded-files/GT48ManagementPremensturalSyndrome.pdf (accessed 6 December 2012).

6 Girman A, Lee R, Kligler B. An integrative medicine approach to premenstrual syndrome. *Am J Obstet Gynecol.* 2003; **188**(5 Suppl): S56–65.

7 Hunter MS, Ussher JM, Cariss M, *et al.* Medical (fluoxetine) and psychological (cognitive-behavioural therapy) treatment for premenstrual dysphoric disorder. A study of treatment processes. *J Psychosom Res.* 2002; **53**(3): 811–17.

8 Freeman EW, Rickels K, Sondheimer SJ, *et al.* A double blind trial of oral progesterone, alprazolam and placebo in treatment of severe premenstrual syndrome. *JAMA.* 1995; **274**(1): 51–7.

9 Landen M, Ericksson O, Sundbland C, *et al.* Compounds with affinity for

serotonergic receptors in the treatment of premenstrual dysphoria: a comparison of buspirone, nefazodone and placebo. *Psychopharmacology.* 2001; **155**(3): 292–8.

10 Wang M, Hammarback S, Lindhe BA, *et al.* Treatment of premenstrual syndrome by spironolactone: a double-blind, placebo-controlled study. *Acta Obstet Gynecol Scand.* 1995; **74**(10): 803–8.

11 Brown J, O'Brien PM, Marjoribanks J *et al.* Selective serotonin reuptake inhibitors for premenstrual syndrome. Cochrane Database Syst Rev. 2009; 2: CD001396.

12 Lopez LM, Kaptein AA, Helmerhorst FM. Oral contraceptives containing drosperinone for premenstrual syndrome. Cochrane Database Syst Rev. 2009; 2: CD006586.

13 Yonkers KA, Brown C, Pearlstein TB, *et al.* Efficacy of a new low-dose oral contraceptive with drospirenone in premenstrual dysphoric disorder. *Obstet Gynecol.* 2005; **106**(3): 492–501.

14 Wyatt K, Dimmock P, Jones P, *et al.* Efficacy of progesterone and progestogens in management of premenstrual syndrome: systematic review. *BMJ.* 2001; 323: 776.

15 Hahn PM, Van Vugt DA, Reid RL. A randomized, placebo-controlled, crossover trial of danazol for the treatment of premenstrual syndrome. *Psychoneuroendocrinology.* 1995; **20**(2): 193–209.

16 Wyatt KM, Dimmock PW, Ismail KM, *et al.* The effectiveness of GnRH with and without 'add-back' therapy in treating premenstrual syndrome: a meta-analysis. *Br J Obstet Gynaecol.* 2004; 111: 585–93.

17 Steege J and Blumenthal J. The effects of aerobic exercise on premenstrual symptoms in middle-aged women: a preliminary study. *J Psychosomatic Res.* 1993; **37**(2): 127–33.

18 Blake F, Salkovskis P, Gath D, *et al.* Cognitive therapy for premenstrual syndrome: a controlled trial. *J Psychosomatic Res.* 1998; **45**(4): 307–18.

3

Menstrual migraine

Migraine is more common in women than in men. Around three out of four people who experience migraines are women. Migraines are most common in women between the ages of 20 to 45 years, perhaps reflecting the various demands – family, social and professional – faced at this stage in life.

A classical migraine headache is usually an intense pain on one, or sometimes both, sides of the head. It is associated with nausea, vomiting, photophobia, spots or flashes of light and sometimes temporary loss of vision.

DEFINITION

Migraine attacks without aura, occurring two days before the onset of menstruation and continuing during the first three days of bleeding in at least two of three menstrual cycles is called menstrual migraine.[1,4] Migraine is defined as episodic headaches lasting between 4 and 72 hours and associated with nausea, vomiting and photophobia.[2]

Menstrual migraines are more severe, last longer, and are more likely to relapse and fail to respond to treatment. They are associated with greater disability as compared to attacks occurring at other times of the menstrual cycle.[5,6,7]

Prevalence

Pure menstrual migraine prevalence is less than 10%.[1,5,10,11] Prevalence is highest in women during the reproductive years of life, affecting 1 in 5 women as compared to 1 in 13 men.[3]

Menstruation itself is a risk factor for migraine without aura in 50%–60% of women.[5,8,9] Women are over 70% more likely to experience migraine in the two days before menstruation and more than 2.5 times more likely to have bad attacks during the first three days of bleed.[4]

Pathophysiology

To understand the pathophysiology it is important to understand the phases of a normal menstrual cycle in response to cyclic hormonal changes.

Gonodotropin-releasing hormone (GnRH):
- stimulates release of FSH and LH, initiating puberty and sustaining menstrual cycle.

Follicle-stimulating hormone (FSH):
- secreted by anterior pituitary gland during the first half of menstrual cycle
- stimulates growth and maturation of the follicle before ovulation
- causes thinning of the endometrium.

Luteinising hormone (LH):
- secreted by the anterior pituitary gland
- stimulates final maturation of follicle
- surge of LH about 14 days before next menstrual period causes ovulation
- stimulates transformation of follicle into corpus luteum
- causes thickening of the endometrium.

Oestrogen:
- secreted primarily by the ovaries, corpus luteum, adrenal cortex and placenta in pregnancy
- stimulates thickening of the endometrium; causes suppression of FSH secretion.

Progesterone:
- secreted by the ovary, corpus luteum and placenta during pregnancy
- inhibits secretion of LH
- increases body temperature
- relaxes smooth muscles and decreases contractions of uterus
- causes cervical secretion of thick mucus
- maintains thickness of endometrium.

Causes of menstrual migraine

During the late luteal phase of a normal menstrual cycle a withdrawal of oestrogen occurs. This is thought to be the cause of menstrual migraine.[7,12] It is also thought to be the cause of headaches during the pill-free interval of the combined contraceptive pill.

Some researchers implicate excessive prostaglandin levels in the blood released by endometrial shedding during menstruation, causing headaches, dysmenorrhoea and heavy bleeds.[13]

Primary care management
History
- Enquire about the timing of an attack. A typical history is an attack starting two days before and continuing during the first three days of the cycle with no attacks at any other time of the cycle.
- Ask about history of aura. The attacks are usually without an aura.
- *Do not rely on history alone.*[14] Encourage use of a 3-month diary to keep a record; this will confirm the diagnosis.
- Enquire about the history of smoking, alcohol and other drugs, e.g. contraceptive pills and medication for allergies.

RED FLAG HEADACHE

- New or unexpected headache.
- Atypical aura (duration > 1 hour).
- Progressive headache worsening over weeks or longer.
- Headache associated with postural change.
- New onset headache in patient with a history of cancer.
- New onset headache in patient with a history of HIV.

Examination
- Routine height, weight, body mass index (BMI), blood pressure and urine check.
- General physical examination and routine eye test to exclude other causes – *refer to an optician if you are not able to do routine eye examinations in your surgery.*

Management
General advice on:
- reduction of alcohol
- reduction of caffeine
- avoiding dehydration
- avoiding missing meals
- avoiding stress.

For acute treatment

Paracetamol

Paracetamol is a good baseline analgesic and is usually well tolerated. Patients might have tried this already and may be seeking advice for a more efficacious therapy. *Remember liver toxicity in overdose.* Use with caution in patients with liver disease, and hepatic or renal impairment.

Codeine, dihydrocodeine

Weak opioids may be useful for some patients. They can cause chronic/severe constipation. Other side effects include nausea, vomiting, confusion and drowsiness, as well as medication-overuse headaches. *Do not add these on repeat prescription and limit the supply to 30 a month.*

TABLE 3.1 Cost-effective prescribing of combined analgesia in primary care (prices from MIMS September 2012) – based on the maximum dose of the cheapest formulation

DRUG	STRENGTH	TABS/CAP/EFF	COST
Co-codamol	8/500 1–2 every 4–6 hrly,max 8 daily	100 tablets	£3.66
Co-codamol	8/500 1–2 every 4–6 hrly, max 8 daily	100 Effer.	£8.02
Co-codamol	15/500 1–2 every 4 hrly, max 8 daily	100 tablets	£8.25
Co-codamol	15/500 1–2 every 4 hrly, max 8 daily	100 Effer.	£8.25
Co-codamol	30/500 1–2 every 4 hrly, max 8 daily	100 tablets	£7,10
Co-codamol	30/500 1–2 every 4 hrly, max 8 daily	100 Effer.	£10.49
Co-dydramol	10/500 1–2 every 4–6 hrly, max 8 daily	100 tablets	£3.56
Dihydrocodeine	30 1 tab every 4–6 hrly	100 tabs	£5.04

Non-steroidal anti-inflammatory drugs (NSAIDs)

NSAIDs work by inhibiting prostaglandins. The main contraindications are asthma, dyspepsia and peptic ulcer. Ibuprofen is traditionally first line with lower risk of gastrointestinal complications than many other NSAIDs.

Ibuprofen has variable patient tolerance and is not effective in menstrual migraine. Naproxen 250 mg TDS or 500 mg twice or three times a day (BD/TDS) peri-menstrually between days (–7 and +6) has shown to be highly effective.[15]

Mefenamic acid 250 mg or 500 mg, three times a day started 2–3 days before the expected onset of period and continued for 2–3 days through the menses can be effective.

An added advantage of mefenamic acid is that it is effective if the patient has symptoms of menorrhagia. *Diclofenac is regarded as a potent NSAID in osteoarthritis and other musculoskeletal pains but not for menstrual migraine – DO NOT USE.*

NSAIDs are effective for menstrual migraine prophylaxis and have the advantage of treating dysmenorrhoea.[16]

TABLE 3.2 Cost-effective prescribing of NSAIDs in primary care (MIMS September 2012) – based on the maximum dose of the cheapest formulation

DRUG	STRENGTH	TABS/CAP	COST
Naproxen	250 mg	56 tabs	£3.34
Naproxen	250 mg EC	56 tabs	£4.29
Naproxen	500 mg	56 tabs	£5.30
Naproxen	500 mg EC	56 tabs	£8.56
Ibuprofen	400 mg	84 tabs	£3.45
Diclofenac	50 mg EC	84 tabs	£1.39
Diclofenac	75 mg EC MR	56 cap	£8.00
Mefenamic acid	250 mg	100 cap	£3.23
Mefenamic acid	500 mg	100 cap	£15.72

Triptans

Of several trials carried out to assess the efficacy of triptans for perimenstrual prophylaxis, the only triptans found to be effective are naratriptan, zolmitriptan, sumatriptan and frovatriptan.[17,18] The most extensive data available covers mainly naratriptan and frovatriptan.

TABLE 3.3 Cost-effective prescribing of triptans in primary care (MIMS September 2012)

DRUG	DOSE	COST
Naratriptan	2.5 mg repeated after at least 4 hours if recurs; max of 5 mg in 24 hours	6 tab pack £24.55
Zolmitriptan	2.5 mg repeated after not less than 2 hours, if recurs; max 10 mg in 24 hours	6 tab pack £18.00 12 tab pack £36.00
Sumatriptan	50 mg repeated after at least 2 hours; max 300 mg in 24 hours	50 mg 6 tab pack £1.61 100 mg 6 tab pack £2.32
Sumatriptan injection	6 mg/0.5 ml 6 mg dose repeated once after at least 1 hour if recurs	2 × 0.5 ml pre-filled syringes and auto injector £42.47

Combined oral contraceptive (COC)

Continuous combined oral pills eliminating the hormonal pill-free interval may be useful in women requiring contraception.[19,20] They should not be used in women who experience migraines with aura because of increased risk of ischaemic stroke.[21] Aura is a focal reversible neurological symptom and can be visual, sensory or motor. It lasts 5–60 minutes before the onset of headache. *If you are unsure, it is generally safest to assume your patient has aura.*

Oestrogen supplements

Transcutaneous oestradiol has been found to be effective for prophylaxis in menstrual migraine in various trials.[22] A dose that achieves a serum oestradiol level of 75 pg/ml has been found to be effective. This can be achieved by using 1.5 mg oestradiol gel or 100 µg oestradiol patch. Some trials have documented an increase in migraine attacks following treatment.[22] Oestrogen supplements are contraindicated in women with a history of deep venous thrombosis, pulmonary embolism and oestrogenic-dependent tumours, similar to COC contraindications.

TABLE 3.4 Cost-effective prescribing in primary care (MIMS September 2012)

Estradiol gel	0.5 mg gel in single dose unit	28	£5.08
Estradiol gel	1 mg gel in single dose unit	28	£5.85
Estradiol gel	0.06% gel, 64 units	80 g pump	£4.80
Estraderm transdermal patch	100 µg/24 hrs	12 patches	£20.70

Progestogen-only contraceptives (POPs)

POPs do not inhibit ovulation and so have little or no role in the management of menstrual migraine. But higher doses (unlicensed) have been shown to be beneficial.[23] *I do not use unlicensed drugs but if you are issuing a prescription, document clearly in the notes.* Irregular bleeds and amenorrhoea are a common side effect.

Levonorgestrel intrauterine system – Mirena coil (IUS)

This works by reducing prostaglandin levels. This method is only useful in women suffering with migraine due to heavy bleeds as this reduces the menstrual flow and the pain.[24] Irregular bleeding is a common reason for discontinuation of this method. The copper coil is not contraindicated but it may cause menstrual headache secondary to dysmenorrhoea and menorrhagia.

TABLE 3.5 Comparative cost as per BNF

Mirena intra-uterine device	Levonorgestrel 52 mg IUS releasing app. 20 µg/24 hrs	1 device £88.00
Nova T 380	Copper wire with silver core on modified plastic T-shaped carrier with monofilament thread	1 device £15.20

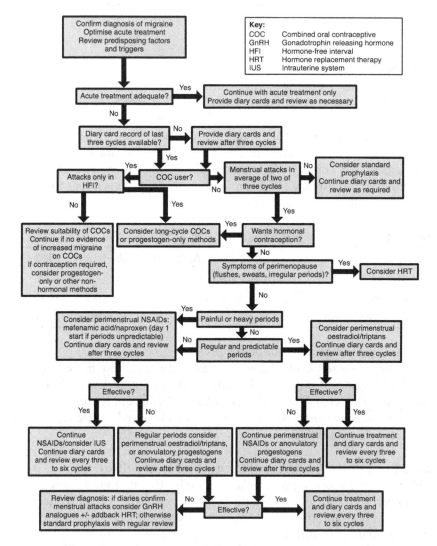

FIGURE 3.1 Flow chart of recommended management of menstrual attacks of migraine

Source: MacGregor EA. Menstrual migraine: a clinical review. *J Fam Plan Reprod Health Care.* 2007; **33**(1): 36–47.

KEY POINTS

- Despite affecting 1 in 7 of the UK population, migraines are underdiagnosed and undertreated.[3]
- The prevalence is highest during the reproductive years of life.
- Menstrual attacks differ from non-menstrual attacks.
- The mainstay of treatment is symptomatic relief of acute attack.
- Non-steroidal anti-inflammatory drugs (NSAIDs) are effective for menstrual migraine prophylaxis and have the advantage of treating dysmenorrhoea.
- Each drug should be trialled for at least 3 months before an alternative is given.

Useful websites

For patients – helplines

Migraine Trust: www.migrainetrust.org

For GPs

British Association for the Study of Headache guidelines: www.bash.org.uk
A diary card can be downloaded from the City of London Migraine Clinic: www.migraineclinic.org.uk

References

1 Dzoljic E, Sipetic S,Vlajinac H, *et al.* Prevalence of menstrually related migraine and nonmigraine primary headaches in female students of Belgrade University. *Headache.* 2001; **42**(3): 185–93.

2 Lipton RB, Dodick D, Sadovsky R, *et al.* A self-administered screener for migraine in primary care: The ID Migraine validation study. *Neurology.* 2003; **61**(3): 375–82.

3 Steiner TJ, Scher AI, Stewart WF, *et al.* The prevalence and disability burden of adult migraine in England and their relationship to age, gender and ethnicity. *Cephalalgia.* 2003; **23**(7): 519–27.

4 MacGregor EA, Hackshaw A. Prevalence of migraine on each day of the menstrual cycle. *Neurology.* 2004; **63**(2): 351–3.

5 MacGregor EA, Brandes J, Eikermann A, *et al.* Impact of migraine on patients and their families: the Migraine And Zolmitriptan Evaluation (MAZE) survey – Phase III. *Curr Med Res Opin.* 2004; **20**(7): 1143–50.

6 Stewart WF, Lipton RB, Chee E, *et al.* Menstrual cycle and headaches in a population sample of migraineurs. *Neurology.* 2005; **55**(10): 1517–33.

7 Pinkerman B, Holroyd K. Menstrual and nonmenstrual migraines differ in women with menstrually-related migraine. *Cephalalgia.* 2010; **30**(10): 1187–94.

8 Granella F, Sances G, Pucci E, *et al.* Migraine with aura and reproductive life events: a case control study. *Cephalalgia.* 2000; **20**(8): 701–7.

9 Wober C, Brannath W, Schmidt K, *et al.* Prospective analysis of factors related to migraine attacks: the PAMINA study. *Cephalalgia.* 2007; **27**(4): 304–14.

10 Granella F, Sances G, Zanferrari C, *et al.* Migraine without aura and reproductive life events: a clinical epidemiological study in 1300 women. *Headache.* 1993; **33**(7): 385–9.

11 MacGregor EA, Chia H, Vohrah RC, *et al.* Migraine and menstruation: a pilot study. *Cephalalgia.* 1990; **10**(6): 305–10.

12 MacGregor EA, Hackshaw A. Prevalence of migraine on each day of the natural menstrual cycle. *Neurology.* 2004; **63**(2): 351–3.

13 Downie J, Poyser N, Wonderlich M. Levels of prostaglandins in human endometrium during normal menstrual cycle. *J Physiol.* 1974; 236: 465–72.

14 MacGregor EA, Isarashi H, Wilkinson M. Headaches and hormones: subjective versus objective assessment. *Headache Quarterly.* 1997; 8: 126–36.

15 Sances G, Martignoni E, Fioroni L, *et al.* Naproxen sodium in menstrual migraine prophylaxis: a double-blind placebo controlled study. *Headache.* 1990; 30(11): 705–9.

16 Mannix LK. Menstrual-related pain conditions: dysmenorrhea and migraine. *J Womens Health (Larchmt).* 2008; **17**(5): 879–91.

17 Silberstein SD, Berner T, Tobin J, *et al.* Scheduled short-term prevention with frovatriptan for migrane occurring exclusively in association with menstruation. *Headache.* 2009; **49**(9): 1283–97.

18 Mannix LK, Savani N, Landy S, *et al.* Efficacy and tolerability of naratriptan for short-term prevention of menstrually related migraine: data from two randomized, double-blind, placebo-controlled studies. *Headache.* 2007; **47**(7): 1037–49.

19 LaGuardia KD, Fisher AC, Bainbridge JD, *et al.* Suppression of estrogen-withdrawal headache with extended transdermal contraception. *Fertil Steril.* 2005; **83**(6): 1875–7.

20 Edelman A, Gallo MF, Nichols MD, *et al.* Continuous versus cyclic use of combined oral contraceptive for contraception: systematic Cochrane review of randomized controlled trials. *Hum Reprod.* 2006; **21**(3): 573–8.

21 World Health Organization. *Medical Eligibility Criteria for Contraceptive Use.* 4th edition. Geneva: WHO; 2009.

22 MacGregor EA, Frith A, Ellis J, *et al.* Prevention of menstrual attacks of migraine: a double-blind placebo-controlled crossover study. *Neurology.* 2006; **67**(12): 2159–63.

23 Davies P, Fursden-Davies C, Rees MC. Progestogens for menstrual migraine. *J Br Menopause Soc.* 2003; **9**(3):134.

24 Crosignani P, Vercellini P, Mosconi P, *et al.* Levonorgestrel-releasing intrauterine device versus hysteroscopic endometrial resection in the treatment of dysfunctional uterine bleeding. *Obstet Gynecol.* 1997; 90: 257–63.

4

Dyspareunia

> **DEFINITION**
>
> Dyspareunia means pain during or after sexual intercourse. Although it can affect men it is more common in women. It can be superficial or deep. Superficial dyspareunia is often localised to vulval or vestibular problems. Deep dyspareunia is often due to pelvic pathology.

Prevalence
It is difficult to estimate the true extent as a lot of women experiencing dyspareunia do not report.

A Swedish survey carried out in 2003 showed a prevalence of 9.3%, with a higher incidence of 6.5% for women aged 50–60 years and 13% for women aged 20–29 years.[1]

Types
Primary dyspareunia: pain since the onset of sexual activity.

Secondary dyspareunia: pain during sexual lifetime.

Causes
- vulvovaginitis
- vaginismus – this is due to involuntary tightness of vagina due to the pubococcygeus muscles
- imperforate hymen (*even though rare but should be remembered*)
- vulval cyst
- herpes simplex virus (HSV)
- lichen sclerosis

- genital psoriasis
- vulval eczema
- vaginitis (infection, chemical irritation, allergy due to spermicides)
- congenital abnormality of the vagina
- inadequate lubrication due to atrophic vaginitis, anxiety/depression, past or present sexual abuse
- vulvodynia
- Bartholin's abscess
- cervicitis
- pelvic inflammatory disease (PID)
- endometriosis
- pelvic mass/ovarian cyst
- uterine causes – fibroid, adenomyosis, fixed retroverted uterus
- irritable bowel/colitis, chronic constipation
- acute or chronic cystitis, interstitial cystitis, urethritis
- incontinence/fear of incontinence
- painful episiotomy scar
- breastfeeding can cause vaginal dryness
- surgery or radiotherapy for malignant disease
- psychosexual causes – mainly trauma caused by sexual abuse
- allergic reaction to spermicides, douches or clothing
- musculoskeletal
- iatrogenic (tamoxifen).

Genital psoriasis

Psoriasis is a multigenic disease affecting 3%–5% of the population. Stress, smoking, beta blockers, chloroquine and lithium are the common trigger factors. Flexural psoriasis typically affects the vulva, especially the mons pubis, the labia majora and genitocrural folds.

Risk factors

- Hysterectomies may be expected to increase the risk but the opposite has also been observed.[2]
- Sexual inexperience.
- The time of menopause.[3]

Primary care management

History

The consultation may be difficult. Remember to consider the emotional aspect of the patient. In most cases a good history will establish the differential diagnosis. Enquire about the following.

- Onset of pain: this will give a clue as to whether dyspareunia is primary or secondary in nature.
- Site of pain: this could establish whether the cause is vulval or pelvic.
- Whether pain is felt with arousal. This could be due to Bartholin's cyst or the hymenal ring band.
- History of pain during penetration (superficial dyspareunia). This could be due to vaginitis or inadequate lubrication (atrophic vaginitis), anxiety/depression, history of sexual abuse.
- History of pain with deep penetration. This could point towards endometriosis, pelvic inflammatory disease, enlarged uterus (fibroid), fixed retroverted (RV) uterus or a pelvic mass.
- History of vulval pain/burning sensation and whether present all the time or only when provoked during sexual intercourse. This goes in favour of vulvodynia.
- Type of pain: sharp or a dull aching pain? Sharp pain may suggest endometriosis. Dull/aching pain may indicate presence of fibroid.
- Any associated symptoms: vaginal discharge, pruritus, vaginal bleeding.
- History of itching with atopy – this may suggest eczema.
- Itching/soreness, with increased vaginal discharge caused by the scales from the plaques – may suggest psoriasis.
- History of temperature: may suggest pelvic inflammatory disease or abscess.
- Any associated symptoms suggestive of menopause – history of hot sweats, flushing of the face and tearing pain during intercourse might suggest atrophic vaginitis.
- History of dysmenorrhoea: pains 2–3 days before the onset of period is a pointer towards endometriosis.
- Urinary symptoms – frequency, urgency or burning. This is suggestive of a urinary tract infection.
- History of breastfeeding – breastfeeding can cause vaginal dryness.
- History of prolapse.
- Medications history: antidepressants, antihypertensives and contraceptive pills can cause vaginal dryness leading to painful intercourse.

Past history
Enquire about:
- obstetric history: difficult forceps, episiotomy, vaginal tears
- history of cancer requiring chemotherapy or radiotherapy which could have caused atrophic vaginitis.

Sexual history

Enquire about:

- past and present sexual activity
- whether the pain precludes all sexual activity
- any history of sexual abuse.

RED FLAG SYMPTOMS

- Temperature
- Pelvic pain
- Abnormal vaginal bleeding
- Vulval abscess

Examination

- Ensure chaperone policy is in place.
- Per abdominal: exclude any abdominal mass and supra pubic tenderness.
- Inspection of external genitalia. Look for:
  — eczema
  — herpes
  — lichen sclerosus
  — psoriatic lesions: typical psoriasis lesions present as symmetrical, pink erythema with smooth edges, well demarcated with a silvery scale. Sometimes the scales may not appear silvery as a result of the moist, humid environment, instead looking beefy red in colour. If margins of the lesions are less well defined, the likely diagnosis is intertrigo, atopic eczema, or lichen simplex
  — fusion of the labia – an unusual presentation of psoriasis
  — genital warts
  — vaginal mucosa: pale vaginal mucosa suggests atrophic vaginitis
  — vaginal discharge.

Pelvic examination

- Exclude any vaginismus: an involuntary contraction of vaginal muscles. In some cases the patient may be unable to abduct her legs, making an internal examination difficult or impossible.
- Exclude imperforate hymen.
- Bimanual examination to exclude fibroids or pelvic mass.
- Observe cervical excitation pain. This suggests pelvic inflammatory disease.
- Record any tenderness in the fornices.

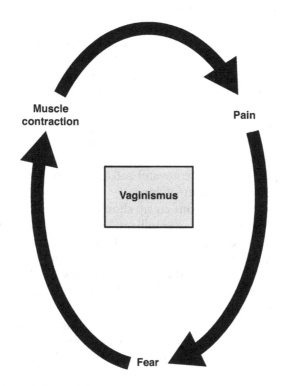

FIGURE 4.1 Pain cycle in vaginismus

Speculum examination
Look for:
- mucopurulent discharge
- cervicitis.

Investigations
In a majority of cases, investigations are not entirely necessary. Consider the following if indicated:
- vaginal swabs if pelvic inflammatory disease is suspected, including chlamydia and gonococcal
- midstream urine (MSU) for culture and sensitivity if symptoms suggestive of cystitis
- pelvic ultrasound to exclude fibroid or a hydrosalpinx.

Management
- Simple reassurance if examination reveals no pain and there is no pathology.

- Advice on simple analgesia and use of different coital positions if the cause is musculoskeletal.
- Vaginal lubricants like KY gel or pelvic relaxation exercises to break the cycle in vaginismus.
- Modification of sexual techniques; increasing the amount of foreplay and delaying penetration will increase vaginal lubrication and decreases dyspareunia.
- Local anaesthetic cream if vulvodynia is suspected.
- Treat vaginal infections depending on the cause.
- For eczema, a non-stinging, potent steroid ointment such as betamethasone valerate (Betnovate) and an oral sedative antihistamine such as hydroxyzine if severe itching.
- For genital psoriasis, aqueous cream should be prescribed both as a soap substitute and as an emollient. Potassium permanganate soaks for 10 minutes twice daily are useful to dry areas of secondary infected skin. Vitamin D analogues such as tacalcitol (Curatoderm) is the primary treatment. Mild or potent topical steroid creams for a short period can be effective. Alphosyl hydrocortisone or clobetasone butyrate 0.05% are usually more effective.
- Restoring the skin's barrier function and reducing inflammation will help to break the itch-scratch cycle in lichen simplex. *Refer these patients to a gynaecologist.* Hydroxyzine or a low-dose amitriptyline can be used to treat itching.
- Active treatment and control of symptoms with an ultra-potent steroid cream is essential to reduce the 3%–5% lifetime risk of squamous cell carcinoma (SCC) associated with lichen sclerosus (LS). *Refer these patients to a gynaecologist/dermatologist.*
- For erosive lichen planus, the treatment of choice is an ultra-potent topical steroid with amitriptyline for pain. Some patients may need systemic treatment initially with hydroxychloroquine, and if necessary followed by a potent immunosuppressant. *These patients are usually under the care of a gynaecologist/dermatologist.*
- Hormone replacement therapy (HRT) if associated with menopausal symptoms and atrophic vaginitis[4] (*exclude HRT contraindications*).
- Psychosexual counselling if vaginismus is the main cause.
- Sildenafil is still under investigation but may be helpful for some cases of arousal problems.[5]

Referral to secondary care

Referral to secondary care may be needed if:
- ultrasound scan shows pelvic pathology, e.g. fibroid, ovarian mass

- if the cause is fixed retroversion – for ventrosuspension
- if tight introitus is the cause – for Fenton's operation
- symptoms and signs are suggestive of endometriosis; this may require laparoscopy
- symptoms are suggestive of colitis or irritable bowel; may need a referral to gastroenterologist
- frequent bouts of cystitis with confirmed bacterial culture and/or incontinence symptoms may need a referral to a urologist.

KEY POINTS

- A physical cause must be excluded before giving a reassurance.
- Treatment should be directed at the underlying cause of dyspareunia.
- Referral to a psychosexual counsellor may be necessary in some cases.

References

1 Danielsson I, Sjoberg I, Stenlund H, *et al*. Prevalence and incidence of prolonged and severe dyspareunia in women: results from a population study. *Scand J Public Health*. 2003; **31**(2): 113–18 (abstract).
2 Rhodes JC, Kjerulff KH, Langenberg PW, *et al*. Hysterectomy and sexual functioning. *JAMA*. 1999; **282**(20): 1934–41 (abstract).
3 Kao A, Binik YM, Kapuscinski A, *et al*. Dyspareunia in postmenopausal women: a critical review. *Pain Res Manag*. 2008 May–June; **13**(3): 243–54 (abstract).
4 Johnston SL, Farrell SA, Bouchard C, *et al*. The detection and management of vaginal atrophy. *J Obstet Gynaecol Can*. 2004 May; **26**(5): 503–15 (abstract).
5 Gregersen N, Jensen PT, Giraldi AE. Sexual dysfunction in the peri- and postmenopause. Status of incidence, pharmacological treatment and possible risks: a secondary publication. *Dan Med Bull*. 2006 Aug 53(3); 349–53 (abstract).

5

Pelvic pain

Most women of reproductive age experience pelvic pains, which may or may not be related to the menstrual cycle.

From a primary care physician perspective, it is important to know the causes of pelvic pain and when to refer/admit a patient. It can be frustrating for both the patients and clinicians who may find it difficult to identify a cause; thus treatment options may by limited.

Aetiology

Gynaecological causes:
- pelvic inflammatory disease (*see* Chapter 9)
- pelvic abscess
- endometriosis (*see* Chapter 19)
- ovarian cyst (torsion, haemorrhage)
- rupture of corpus luteum cyst
- ovulation mittelschmerz (German: 'middle pain') – ovulation pain is unilateral pelvic pain; the pain is usually mid-cycle and short lasting
- fibroid degeneration – fibroids can cause acute pain if they degenerate; this is common in pregnancy
- prolapse
- ovarian hyperstimulation syndrome
- pelvic cancer
- pelvic vein thrombosis.

Non-gynaecological causes:
- urinary tract infection
- appendicitis
- renal colic
- irritable bowel syndrome

- constipation
- diverticulitis
- bowel obstruction
- strangulated hernia
- ectopic pregnancy
- miscarriage
- uterine rupture
- adhesions due to previous surgery
- postherpetic neuralgia
- psychological and social issues.

Types

Acute pelvic pain

Pelvic pain that comes on suddenly for the first time is called acute pelvic pain. The common causes of acute pelvic pain in women who are not pregnant are:

- pelvic inflammatory disease
- urinary tract infection
- ovarian cyst torsion or rupture
- pelvic abscess
- endometriosis – a rare cause.

Chronic pelvic pain

Intermittent or constant pelvic pain in the lower abdomen or pelvis of at least 6 months in duration, not occurring exclusively with menstruation or sexual intercourse, is chronic pelvic pain. Chronic pain is usually more severe and lasts for a longer period of time. It presents in primary care at a rate of 38 per 1000 women every year, comparable to asthma at 37 per 1000 and back pain at 41 per 1000.[1] It can impact on a woman's ability to function.[2] The common causes are:

- endometriosis: the cardinal symptoms of dysmenorrhoea, dyspareunia and chronic pelvic pain are characteristic of endometriosis or adenomyosis[3]
- fibroids
- prolapse: pelvic organ prolapse can be a cause of pain[6]
- recurrent urinary tract infection
- chronic interstitial cystitis: in three observational studies of women with chronic pelvic pain presenting to secondary care, 38%–84% had symptoms suggestive of interstitial cystitis[4,5]
- irritable bowel syndrome, diverticular disease
- ovarian cyst

- adhesions: caused by endometriosis, previous surgery or previous infection
- pelvic congestion
- musculoskeletal: pain may arise from the joints in the pelvis or from damage to the muscles in the abdominal wall or pelvic floor
- pelvic inflammatory disease – a rare cause
- pudendal nerve damage or entrapment
- no organic cause found at laparoscopy in at least 33% of cases.[7]

Primary care management

Any patient complaining of pelvic pain must be seen on the same day by a GP. A thorough history and examination will differentiate between women requiring urgent admission and those who can be managed in the community.

History

Pelvic pain is a symptom rather than a diagnosis. A good history and an examination are essential to reach a diagnosis and to prevent an unnecessary referral to secondary care. History must include not only gynaecological but also urinary or bowel symptoms.

- Enquire about history of pain: site of pain (pelvic or lower abdominal pain), nature of pain, radiation (shoulder tip pain). A pain originating from the uterus, fallopian tubes or ovaries is usually in the middle of the lower abdomen. Pain that is more to one side is due to an ovarian cause. Ask whether the pain is associated with sexual intercourse; a history of pain during sexual intercourse is due to endometriosis.
- Enquire about whether the pain is acute (sudden or unsuspected) or chronic (recurrent).
- Ask about the nature of the pain and any aggravating or relieving factors. A history of burning, aching or shooting pain that is worse on sitting and relieved on standing or lying flat is *probably due to pudendal nerve entrapment – a rare cause.* Pain made worse by standing, menstruation or sexual intercourse is probably due to pelvic congestion.
- Enquire about relationship with menstrual cycle. Pelvic pain which varies markedly over the menstrual cycle is likely to be due to endometriosis.
- Enquire as to the last menstrual bleed, any history of amenorrhoea or abnormal vaginal bleeding (intermenstrual or post-coital).
- Any history of fainting or dizziness.
- Any history of time off work or avoiding activities.

- Get a detailed history of urinary symptoms – frequency, urgency or blood-stained urine.
- Enquire about any history of temperature. High temperature, back pains and urinary symptoms may be a pointer to pyelonephritis.
- Ask if any bowel symptoms – constipation/diarrhoea, colicky/dull pain, bloating, change in bowel frequency, pain or discomfort relieved by defecation, mucus in the stool, bloating, fresh bleeding per rectum or black motions.
- Enquire about any symptoms suggestive of depression, anxiety and sleep disorders.
- If suspecting sexual abuse, this must be asked with great sensitivity. Remember this could be a *cause of chronic pelvic pain.*[8]

Examination

General physical:
- pallor
- pulse
- blood pressure.

Tachycardia and hypotension are late signs of shock in young women who can loose > 1500 ml of blood before there is a change in clinical condition.

Per abdominal:
Examine the abdomen and look for any:
- distension
- guarding
- tenderness
- rigidity.

Tenderness at sacroiliac joints or the symphysis pubis is suggestive of a musculoskeletal cause of pain.

Pelvic examination

This is not necessary in a majority of cases unless pelvic inflammatory disease is suspected. *In these patients remember to do pelvic swabs before initiating the treatment.*

RED FLAG SIGNS AND SYMPTOMS

- Acutely unwell patient
- Rapid onset of severe symptoms – pain, vomiting, tenderness and temperature
- Bleeding per rectum
- New bowel symptoms over the age of 50 years
- Pelvic mass
- Excessive weight loss
- Post-coital bleeding
- New pain after the menopause
- Suicidal ideation
- Suspicion of ectopic pregnancy or acute appendicitis
- Suspected haemorrhage, torsion or ruptured ovarian cyst
- Suspected or confirmed ovarian tumour.

Red flag signs and symptoms in women with chronic pelvic pain ⚑

- Rectal bleeding
- New bowel symptoms in women aged >50 years
- New pain after menopause
- Pelvic mass

- Suicidal ideation
- Excessive weight loss
- Irregular vaginal bleeding in women aged >40 years
- Post-coital bleeding

Source: Royal College of Obstetricians and Gynaecologists. Chronic pelvic pain, initial management. Green-top guideline 41. RCOG Press; 2005.

⚑ *indicates a potentially serious condition that should not be ignored*

FIGURE 5.1 Red flag signs and symptoms in women with chronic pelvic pain

Investigations

- Urine analysis: send mid-stream urine for culture and sensitivity (MSU) if indicated.
- Pregnancy test to exclude ectopic pregnancy. For any woman of childbearing age presenting with abdominal pain, pregnancy should be excluded by *checking the serum β-hCG in the presence of a negative qualitative urine test.*
- Beta-human chorionic gonadotrophin (hCG). A single test is of limited value in confirming ectopic pregnancy. Tests taken 48 hours apart are needed to confirm the diagnosis.

- Triple swabs to screen pelvic infection.
- Full blood count if suspecting pelvic infection. The white blood cell (WBC) count will be raised.
- Erythrocyte sedimentation rate (ESR) and C-reactive protein (CRP) (markers of inflammation). They are useful to monitor the response to therapy.
- Cancer antigen 125 (CA125) if suspecting ovarian cancer. Persistent or frequent symptoms (more than 12 times per month), e.g. bloating, early satiety, urinary frequency, pelvic pain *particularly in women over the age of 50 years.*
- Transvaginal or trans-abdominal ultrasound scan. It is of limited value when investigating pelvic pain but should be performed if suspected ovarian pathology.
- Diagnostic laparoscopy if suspecting an ovarian or uterine pathology. Fifty per cent of laparoscopies are negative.
- Magnetic resonance imaging (MRI). Transvaginal scanning and MRI are useful tests to diagnose adenomyosis. A systematic review of 14 trials examining the diagnostic accuracy of transvaginal scans for diagnosing adenomyosis found a sensitivity of 82.5% and specificity of 84.6%.[9]
- Venography or magnetic resonance imaging (MRI) if suspected pelvic congestion to image the varicosities.
- Urological investigation – cystoscopy if urological cause is suspected.
- Sigmoidoscopy/colonoscopy/barium enema if persisting bowel symptoms.
- Hospital anxiety and depression score (HADS) or patient's health questionnaire (PHQ-9) if suspecting anxiety or depression.

Treatment

After a proper history and examination decide whether the patient needs a hospital admission or can be managed within primary care. A large proportion of women can be managed by their GP.

Treatment depends on the cause. Empirical use of strong analgesia and antibiotic without confirming the diagnosis must be avoided.

- Conservative treatment is all that is needed if pain is caused by a degenerate fibroid.
- Completing a daily pain diary for 2–3 months and focussing on the menstrual cycle may be useful in understanding the cause of pain. Simple analgesia include regular paracetamol and non-steroidal anti-inflammatory drugs (NSAIDs). If prescribing opioids, the risk of addiction must be carefully considered.
- Consider hormonal contraception to prevent ovulation if pain is

secondary to ovulation. The levonorgestrel-releasing intrauterine system (Mirena coil) could be considered.[10]

- Ovarian suppression with combined oral contraceptive pill (COC), progestogens, danazol or GnRH analogues can be an effective treatment for pain due to endometriosis.[11] If suspected residual ovary syndrome, trapped ovary and pelvic congestion, a trial of ovarian suppression should be given before embarking on hysterectomy. Use of danazol or a GnRH agonist should be limited to 6 months because of the adverse effect on bone mineral density. If necessary, tibolone can be given as 'add-back' therapy.
- If the cause is pelvic inflammatory disease, *see* Chapter 9.
- Oophorectomy is needed if the diagnosis is ovarian torsion or haemorrhage. An ultrasound scan can show features suggestive of torsion.[12]
- If suspected ectopic pregnancy, follow the map of medicine pathway (*see* Figure 5.2).
- If the history suggests a non-gynaecological cause of pain, referral to a urologist, gastroenterologist, physiotherapist, psychologist or psychosexual counsellor should be considered.
- Dietary advice and a trial of antispasmodics to women with irritable bowel syndrome. Referral to a dietician may be necessary in some patients.
- Laxatives may be prescribed if simple measures such as increasing fluid intake, dietary fibre and physical exercise fail to improve symptoms of

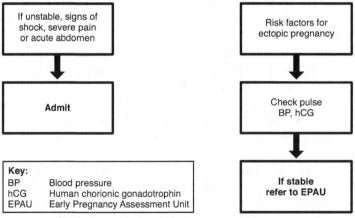

FIGURE 5.2 Pathway for suspected ectopic pregnancy
Source: Based on Map of Medicine. Ectopic pregnancy: www.mapofmedicine.com

constitution. Possibility of iatrogenic causes of constipation (such as opioid) must be remembered, especially over-the-counter medicaments (OTCs).

- Any change in bowel habit must be investigated and the patient referred if there are red flag symptoms.

TABLE 5.1 Key features of agents most commonly used for mild to moderate pain management

KEY FEATURES OF AGENTS MOST COMMONLY USED FOR MILD TO MODERATE PAIN MANAGEMENT		
NON-NSAID AGENTS		
ANALGESIC	KEY CHARACTERISTICS	COMMENTS
Paracetamol	Good baseline analgesia and well tolerated, but rarely used (patients have often tried it before seeking medical advice and are looking for more efficacious therapy).	Liver toxicity in overdose. Use with caution in patients with alcoholic liver disease, hepatic or renal impairment.
Codeine, dihydrocodeine	Weak opioids	Can cause chronic/severe constipation; most suitable for acute pain. Nausea, vomiting, drowsiness and confusion limit value. Side effects magnified with dihydrocodeine therapy.
NSAID AGENTS		
	KEY CHARACTERISTICS	COMMENTS
Ibuprofen	Traditional first-line. Lower risk of gastrointestinal complications than many other NSAIDs.	Variable patient tolerance. Four-dose regimen difficult for those on concomitant medication.
Diclofenac	Widely prescribed and regarded as a potent NSAID. Effective for osteoarthritis or other musculoskeletal pain that is uncontrolled with weaker agents. Not effective for pelvic pain.	Gastrointestinal side effects (dyspepsia and irritation). Modified-release formulations are costly.
Naproxen	Low-cost generic agent for osteoarthritis and acute musculoskeletal pain. Not effective for pelvic pain.	Severe gastrointestinal side effects. Possible increased risk of cardiovascular events with long-term, high-dose use [The Food and Drug Administration (FDA) statement, 20.12.04]
Mefenamic acid	Useful in mild to moderate pain, dysmenorrhoea and menorrhagia.	Gastrointestinal side effects. Rarely hypotension and haemolytic anaemia.

- If suspected interstitial cystitis, uro-gynaecologist input is needed.
- Options for treatment of pudendal nerve entrapment include local anaesthetic injections or a trial of gabapentin or amitriptyline.
- Transcutaneous electronic nerve stimulation (TENS) or acupuncture in rare cases.
- If suspected pelvic congestion, treatment may include NSAIDs, ovarian suppression, embolisation or hysterectomy with bilateral oophorectomy.
- Division of dense vascular adhesions should be considered for pain relief. In a randomised controlled trial, 48 women with chronic pelvic pain underwent laparotomy with or without division of adhesions. Although overall no difference was noted between the two groups, a subset analysis showed that division of dense, vascular adhesions produced significant pain relief.[13] There is no evidence to support the division of fine adhesions in women with chronic pelvic pain.
- Co-existing anxiety/depression should be managed appropriately with anxiolytics or antidepressants.
- Referral to a pain clinic can be helpful when all management options are exhausted.

KEY POINTS

- A pregnancy test is a MUST for any woman of reproductive age with acute pelvic pain.
- In a woman of childbearing age presenting with abdominal pain, pregnancy should be excluded by checking the serum β-hCG in the presence of a negative qualitative urine test.
- A good history and examination can decide whether hospitalisation is needed.
- Many women with chronic pelvic pain can be managed within primary care.
- Pelvic ultrasound is not the first-line investigation unless ovarian pathology is suspected.
- Fifty per cent of the diagnostic laparoscopies are negative.
- Rapid onset of severe symptoms, suspicion of ectopic pregnancy or acute appendicitis represents an emergency and the patient MUST be admitted.
- White cell count and C-reactive protein have a limited value in diagnosis. They are useful to monitor the response to therapy.
- Enquiry should be made regarding social and psychological issues, which commonly occur in patients with chronic pelvic pain.

Useful websites

For patients – helplines

Ectopic Pregnancy Trust: www.ectopic.org.uk

Miscarriage Association: www.miscarriageassociation.org.uk

Pelvic pain support network: www.pelvicpain.org.uk

Royal College of Obstetricians and Gynaecologists. Long-term pelvic pain: information for you: www.rcog.org.uk/womens-health/clinical-guidance/long-term-pelvic-pain-information-you

Royal College of Obstetricians and Gynaecologists. Patient leaflets on acute pelvic inflammatory disease, ectopic pregnancy, bleeding and pain in early pregnancy: www.rcog.org.uk/womens-health/patient-information

For GPs

Royal College of Obstetricians and Gynaecologists. Development of RCOG Green-top guidelines: producing a clinical practice guideline. www.rcog.org.uk/womens-health/clinical-guidance/development-rcog-green-top-guidelines-producing-clinical-practice-gu

References

1 Zondervan KT, Yudkin PL, Vassey MP, *et al*. Prevalence and incidence of chronic pelvic pain in primary care: evidence from a national general practice database. *Br J Obstet Gynaecol*. 1999; **106**(11): 1149–55.

2 Grace V, Zondervan K. Chronic pelvic pain in women in New Zealand: comparative well-being, comorbidity and impact on work and other activities. *Health Care Women Int*. 2006; **27**(7): 585–99.

3 Scialli AR. Evaluating chronic pelvic pain. A consensus recommendation. Pelvic Pain Expert Working Group. *J Reprod Med*. 1999; **44**(11): 945–52.

4 Clemons JL, Arya LA, Myers DL. Diagnosing interstitial cystitis in women with chronic pelvic pain. *Obstet Gynecol*. 2002; 100: 337–41.

5 Reddy J, Barber MD, Walters MD, *et al*. Lower abdominal and pelvic pain with advanced pelvic organ prolapse: a case-control study. *Am J Obstet Gynecol*. 2011; **204**(6): 537 e1–5.

6 Montenegro ML, Gomide LB, Mateus-Vasconcelos EL, *et al*. Abdominal myofascial pain syndrome must be considered in the differential diagnosis of chronic pelvic pain. *Eur J Obstet Gynecol Reprod Biol*. 2009; **147**(1): 21–4.

7 Danielj JP, Khan KS. Chronic pelvic pain in women. *BMJ*. 2010 Oct 5; 341: c4834.

8 Raphael KG, Widom CS, Lange G. Childhood victimization and pain in adulthood: a prospective investigation. *Pain*. 2001; **92**(1–2): 283–93.

9 Bazot M, Cortez A, Darai E, *et al*. Ultrasonography compared with magnetic resonance imaging for the diagnosis of adenomyosis: correlation with histopathology. *Hum Reprod*. 2001; **16**(11): 2427–33.

10 Aslam N, Blunt S, Latthe P. Effectiveness and tolerability of levonorgestrel intrauterine system in adolescents. *J Obstet Gynaecol.* 2010; **30**(5): 489–91.

11 Royal College of Obstetricians and Gynaecologists. The investigation and management of endometriosis. Green-top Guideline No 24. London: RCOG; 2008. Available at: www.rcog.org.uk/womens-health/clinical-guidance/investigation-and-management-endometriosis-green-top-24 (accessed 6 December 2012).

12 Webb EM, Green GE, Scoutt LM. Adnexal mass with pelvic pain. *Radiol Clin North Am.* 2004; **42**(2): 329–48.

13 Swank DJ, Swank-Bordewijk SC, Hop WC, *et al.* Laparoscopic adhesiolysis in patients with chronic abdominal pain: a blinded randomised controlled multicentre trial. *Lancet.* 2003; **361**(9365): 1247–51.

6

Vaginal dryness

The average menopausal age in the UK is 52 years, at which point a woman's ovaries stop producing oestrogen. It is the lack of oestrogen that causes vaginal dryness. Vaginal dryness can affect over half of postmenopausal women aged between 51–60 years. If a woman experiences menopause under the age of 40 years it is known as premature menopause.[3] This could be due to ovarian failure or post hysterectomy.

Prevalence

About 58% of postmenopausal women experience vaginal dryness. About 17% of women aged 18–50 years experience problems with vaginal dryness during sex even before they reach menopause.[1] In observational studies 27% to 55% of postmenopausal women reported vaginal dryness[2] and 19% reported irritation or itching.

Causes

Vaginal dryness can be caused by:
- infrequent sexual intercourse
- menopause or perimenopause
- psychological factors
- anxiety and/or depression
- vaginismus
- post hysterectomy
- premature ovarian failure – hypothyroidism, Addison's disease, Turner's syndrome, Down's syndrome, radiotherapy or chemotherapy
- Sjögren's syndrome (can also cause dry eyes and dry mouth)
- postnatal
- breastfeeding

- alcohol
- drugs such as thiazides, spironolactone, sedatives and tranquillisers
- injuries to spinal cord
- multiple sclerosis
- diabetes mellitus
- tuberculosis (TB), mumps (rare causes) – can cause premature ovarian failure.

Primary care management

Vaginal dryness can cause emotional, psychological and relationship problems. It takes a lot of courage for a woman to seek help. She may be tearful during consultation and a sympathetic approach is required. *These patients may need to book a double appointment.*

History

Enquire about history of:

- duration of symptoms and any associated pain, irritation or burning of vagina or vulva
- postcoital bleeding or spotting
- any associated menopausal symptoms
- history of vaginal discharge
- any associated urinary symptoms
- detailed sexual history – sexual partners, frequency of sexual intercourse
- any symptoms suggestive of anxiety or depression
- medication history of prescribed or over-the-counter drugs.

Examination

This is not necessary in the majority of patients. Usually examination is difficult and smear-taking can be painful and uncomfortable.

- Inspection: to exclude any vulval or vaginal pathology.
- Per vaginal (PV) examination to exclude any pelvic pathology.
- Perform smear if patient is due for one.

Investigations

Complete a urine test if there are associated urinary symptoms.

Treatment

Too many women think vaginal dryness is an unavoidable part of growing older and may not talk about it freely. It should be managed as any other condition.

- Some women seek reassurance that this is a part of growing old. In these cases explain the nature of the problem and offer general advice.
- General advice: avoid perfumed soaps, bubble baths, vinegar, yoghurt or other douches, hand lotions or any over-the-counter (OTC) lubricants. Advise the patient to take time during sexual intercourse.
- Non-hormonal lubricants: these are effective in relieving symptoms of pruritus, irritation and dyspareunia, and restoring acidic vaginal pH levels.[4]
- Low-dose oestrogen: used locally this can be highly effective.[5] Vaginal administration of oestrogens improves the quality of the vaginal epithelium in atrophic vaginitis and relieves the associated symptoms of irritation, pruritus and dyspareunia. There is also limited evidence that it may protect against recurrent urinary tract infections[6] and relieve urethral syndrome and urgency.[7]
- These beneficial effects are achieved through actions on collagen metabolism and restoration of an acidic vaginal pH.[8] A Swedish epidemiological case-control study found that exclusive use of low-dose vaginal oestrogen preparations among 297 users for 5 years or more was not associated with a significant increase in relative risk for endometrial cancer or atypical endometrial hyperplasia.[9]
- The main advantage of a vaginal preparation is that oestrogen is delivered directly to the site of symptoms with no systemic absorption. Pharmacokinetic studies have shown that vaginally administered oestrogens undergo less metabolism by the liver as compared to orally administered formulations.
- To obtain a desired plasma concentration, a lower dose of vaginally administered formulation is required as compared to an oral dose. Oestriol administered vaginally produces a similar plasma level to that of a 20-times higher dose administered orally.[10]
- Although small increases in serum oestradiol have been reported in some studies using vaginal oestriol or conjugated equine oestrogens cream, this has not been seen in studies of vaginal oestradiol tablets or rings.[11]
- Treatment should be reviewed at least annually with special consideration given to symptoms of endometrial hyperplasia or carcinoma. If vaginal bleeding occurs during long-term treatment with vaginal oestrogens, the treatment must be stopped and *an urgent 2-week referral* must be done for assessment of endometrial thickness and biopsy.
- Oral hormone replacement therapy (HRT): HRT can be prescribed for distressing menopausal symptoms or premature menopause, provided there are no absolute contraindications.

TABLE 6.1 Cost-effective topical oestrogens

Gynest intravaginal cream Most cost-effective to prescribe	Estriol 0.01% 80 gm with applicator	£4.67
Ovestin intravaginal cream	Estriol 0.1% 15 gm with applicator	**£4.45**
Ortho-Gynest pessaries	Estriol 500 ug 15 pessaries	£4.73
Vaginal ring (Estring)	Releasing estradiol Approximately 7.5 ug/24 hours	1 ring pack £31.42
Non-hormonal vaginal treatments – Hyalofemme	30 g tube with reusable applicator	£4.60
Non-hormonal vaginal treatments – Repadina ovules	10 ovules	£8.14
Non-hormonal vaginal treatments – Replens MD	3-dose pack	£3.65
	6-dose pack	£5.89
	35 g pack (up to 12 applications) plus applicator	£5.89
Sylk	40 gms, sufficient for 75 to 100 applications	£5.16

Vaginal cream to be inserted, one applicator daily and preferably in the evening until improvement occurs, reducing to one applicator twice a week for a maximum period of 3–6 months.

Vaginal pessary to be inserted, one pessary daily, preferably in the evening until improvement occurs. Maintenance dose is one pessary twice a week, for a maximum period of 3–6 months.

Vaginal ring is inserted in to upper third of vagina and worn continuously. This is replaced after 3 months. Maximum duration of treatment is 2 years.

Hyalofemme – once every 3 days.

Repadina – one vaginal ovule nightly until symptoms are controlled, then used as required.

Replens MD – one application 3 times weekly in the morning.

Sylk – use as required.

KEY POINTS

- Vaginal dryness can have a detrimental effect on women's psychological and emotional well-being.
- Non-hormonal lubricants are effective in relieving symptoms of pruritus, irritation and dyspareunia.
- Low-dose vaginal oestrogens in postmenopausal women are effective in alleviating symptoms of atrophic vaginitis and possibly in preventing recurrent urinary tract infections.
- Topical oestrogens should be used in the smallest effective amount to minimise systemic side effects.

- An urgent 2-week referral must take place if vaginal bleeding occurs during treatment with vaginal oestrogens.

Useful websites

For patients – helplines

Menopause Information—Concerned about Menopause? www.symptomfind.com/Menopause.

Women's Health Concern: www.womens-health-concern.org/help/focuson/focus_vaginaldryness.html

For GPs

Bacterial vaginosis: Bacterial Vaginosis BASHH. www.bash.org/documents/62/62.pdf. National Guideline For The Management of Bacterial Vaginosis (2006) Clinical Effectiveness Group. British Association For Sexual Health And HIV.

Candida: National Guideline on the Management of Vulvovaginal Candidiasis www.bashh.org/documents/50/50.pdf

Treatment advice: Health Protection Agency website, Vaginal discharge. Reviewed and updated July 2011 Vaginal Discharge Vaginitis-Quick Ref Guide (PDF) www.hpa.org.uk/infections/topics_az/primary_care_guidance/menu.htm

References

1 Laumann EO, Paik A, Rosen RC. Sexual dysfunction in the United States: prevalence and predictors. *JAMA*. 1999; **281**(6): 537–44.
2 Dennerstein L, Dudley EC, Hopper JL *et al.* A prospective population based study of menopausal symptoms. *Obstet Gynecol.* 2000; **96**(3): 351–8.
3 Hendrix SL. Bilateral oophorectomy and premature menopause. *Am J Med.* 2005; **118**(12B): 131S–135S.
4 Bygdeman M, Swahn ML. Replens versus dienoestrol cream in the symptomatic treatment of vaginal atrophy in postmenopausal women. *Maturitas.* 1996; **23**(3): 259–63.
5 Cardozo L, Bachmann G, McClish D, *et al.* Meta analysis of oestrogen therapy in the management of urogenital atrophy in postmenopausal women: second report of the Hormones and Urogenital Committee. *Obstet Gynecol.* 1998; 92: 722–7.
6 Eriksen B. A randomised, open, parallel group study on the preventative effect of an oestradiol-releasing vaginal ring (Estring) on recurrent urinary tract infections in postmenopausal women. *Am J Obstet Gynecol.* 1999; **180**(5): 1072–9.
7 Hillard T. Principles of hormone replacement therapy: part 1. *Trends Urol Gynaecol Sex Health.* 2000; 5: 22–7.
8 Jackson S, Janes M, Abrams P. The effect of oestradiol on vaginal collagen metabolism in postmenopausal women with genuine stress incontinence. *Br J Obstet Gynaecol.* 2002; 109: 339–44.

9 Weiderpass E, Baron JA, Adami HO, *et al.* Low-potency oestrogen and risk of endometrial cancer: a case-control study. *Lancet.* 1999; **353**(9167): 1824–8.

10 Kuhl H. Pharmacokinetics of oestrogens and progestogens. *Maturitas.* 1990; **12**(3): 171–97.

11 Nachtigall LE. Clinical trial of the estradiol vaginal ring in the US. *Maturitas.* 1995; 22 Suppl: S43.

7

Vulvodynia

DEFINITION

Vulvodynia is defined by the International Society for the Study of Vulvovaginal Disease (ISSVD) as vulval discomfort occurring in the absence of any visible findings or a specific clinically identifiable neurological disorder. It is a chronic neurogenic pain syndrome.[1]

Prevalence

Women of all ages, races or socio-economic groups can suffer from vulvodynia. Prevalence is not known but a recent population based survey from the United States found that 16% of women experienced knife like/chronic burning vulval pain that lasted at least three months or longer and nearly 7% were symptomatic at the time of survey.[2] It is a highly distressing condition.

Aetiology

Vulvodynia is still a poorly understood condition. There are several theories about the aetiology *but no evidenced-based cause or causes are known at the time of writing.* Genetic susceptibility, hormonal factors and infections have been thought to be some of the aetiological factors.

It is not clear whether anxiety or depression is the cause or effect, but it certainly coexists with vulvodynia.

Categories:

a) provoked – burning pain on sexual intercourse, per speculum examination or insertion of tampon

b) unprovoked – pain brought on by tight clothes, prolonged sitting or cycling

c) mixed.

Provoked:
a) common in the reproductive age
b) precipitated by penetration, sexual intercourse, tampons and speculum examination.

Unprovoked:
a) common in menopausal age
b) precipitated by prolonged sitting, cycling, tight clothing and penetration.

Classification

International Society for the Study of Vulvovaginal Disease (ISSVD) classification of vulval pain:

A Vulval pain related to a specific disorder:
  1. Pelvic infections – candidiasis, herpes.
  2. Dermatological – lichen planus, lichen sclerosis.
  3. Neoplastic – squamous cell carcinoma, Paget's disease.
  4. Neurological – spinal nerve compression, herpes neuralgia.
B Vulvodynia:
  1. Generalised: provoked (sexual, non-sexual or both)unprovoked mixed (provoked and unprovoked).
  2. Localised: provoked (sexual, non-sexual or both) unprovoked mixed (provoked and unprovoked).

Vestibulodynia

Provoked pain localised to the vestibule region with pain experienced on sexual and non-sexual touch is called vestibulodynia. The maximal area of tenderness is over the entrance to the Bartholin's glands.[3]

Primary care management

History

A good history can help early diagnosis, early management and appropriate referral if indicated. This is important for women to regain control of their lives. The age of the patient will give you a clue as to whether vulvodynia is provoked or unprovoked.

  Enquire about:
• the nature of the pain (irritating, stinging or sharp), any associated itching, history of back pain

- any relieving factors; pain relieved by standing or lying flat is probably due to pudendal neuralgia
- history of white spots (shiny itchy spots on the vulva in a middle-aged woman, spreading to whole of vulva and/or anal skin may suggest lichen sclerosus)
- exact anatomical site of the pain, e.g. hemivulvodynia, generalised vulvodynia or clitorodynia
- triggers of pain, e.g. penetration, tampons, prolonged sitting, cycling or sexual intercourse
- past history of obstetric trauma
- past or present history of vulval itch or vulval skin problems
- any relevant medical history such as diabetes or thyroid
- history of any skin problems such as eczema or psoriasis
- history of dyspareunia
- any symptoms suggestive of anxiety/depression or social isolation
- any previous treatments and how long they were used for
- history of past or present sexual abuse
- psychosexual issues – past or present.

Examination

In most cases examination is usually normal with no visible findings, however a proper examination must be carried out.

- Vulval inspection to exclude infection, malignancy or dermatological cause. Check for any erythema in the vestibule.
- Look for shiny spots/white areas, splitting or cracking of the skin.
- Observe any tension of the pelvic floor muscles. This could be due to reflex response to examination. Gentle examination with one finger is often useful.
- Light touch with a cotton bud in the vestibule may reveal marked hypersensitivity and pain.

Investigations

Not needed routinely but if clinically indicated carry out:

- vaginal swabs if infection is suspected
- full blood count to exclude anaemia
- fasting blood sugar to exclude diabetes
- thyroid function test (TFT) if suspecting thyroid dysfunction
- biopsy of the affected skin if lichen sclerosus is suspected.

Treatment

The treatment depends on the cause. However, most vulval problems can

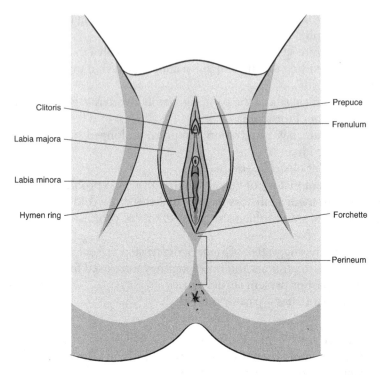

Clitoris

Labia majora

Labia minora

Hymen ring

Prepuce

Frenulum

Forchette

Perineum

FIGURE 7.1 Normal anatomy of vulva

be managed within primary care. Reassurance is important. The aim of the treatment is to minimise the symptoms and to help the patient lead as normal a life as possible. Treatment must be individualised, involving the patient in the management.[4]

- Advice about vulval skin care. Good vulval skin care is important. Avoiding perfumed soaps, sprays and bubble baths can be beneficial. Massaging vulval skin with emollients like Diprobase cream may help to desensitise the hypersensitive area.
- Use of emollient cream or ointment instead of soap to clean the affected area.
- Refer the patient to a gynaecologist/dermatologist if suspecting lichen sclerosis. Steroid cream or ointment if lichen sclerosis is diagnosed *as advised by the specialist*. This eases the irritation but may take about 3 months of treatment for the skin to look and feel better.
- The British Association of Dermatologists has produced evidence-based guidance on the management of lichen sclerosus that includes the use of ultra-potent topical corticosteroids and emollients.[6]
- Cancer of the vulva is an uncommon complication of lichen sclerosis.

Teach the patient to get into the habit of using a hand-held mirror to check the vulva once a month and feel the skin with their fingers.

- Local anaesthetic cream like lidocaine 5% ointment or 2% gel used before sexual intercourse or more often during the day, may be useful for some patients.
- Prescribe an antifungal if the diagnosis is vulvovaginal candidiasis. Guidelines for the management of acute and chronic candidiasis have been developed by the British Association for Sexual Health and HIV.[5]
- Topical oestrogens may help some postmenopausal women with unprovoked vulvodynia.
- Acupuncture or transcutaneous electrical nerve stimulation (TENS) machine can be useful in some selected patients.
- Systemic medication – tricyclic antidepressants like amitriptyline or nortriptyline, starting at a lower dose and titrating the dose as per response. Start amitriptyline at 10 mg daily at night, gradually increasing to a maximum of 75 mg daily. The most common side effects are nausea, vomiting, taste disturbance, tinnitus, dry mouth, blurred vision, constipation, agitation, confusion and drowsiness. The patient should be encouraged to persist with treatment, as some tolerance seems to develop with time. Remember to prescribe limited quantities because of cardiovascular and epileptogenic side effects in over-dosage.
- Women with a poor response or low toleration to amitriptyline may try anticonvulsants – gabapentin or pregabalin. Remember *gabapentin is more cost-effective*. Start gabapentin 300 mg once daily on day 1, increasing to 300 mg twice daily on day 2, then 300 mg three times daily on day 3; **OR** 300 mg three times daily on day 1, then increased according to response in steps of 300 mg (in three divided doses) every 2–3 days up to a maximum of 3.6 gm daily. Pregabalin is started at 150 mg daily in 2–3 divided doses, increasing to 300 mg daily after 3–7 days to a maximum of 600 mg in two or three divided doses. Women started on these medications must be reviewed every 6 months.
- Surgical excision of the vestibule (vestibulectomy) may benefit a minority of patients with provoked pain. Surgery should not be the first-line treatment for women with provoked vulvodynia, and those who undergo surgery will need psychosexual support pre- and postoperatively.[7] Modified vestibulectomy, in which a horseshoe-shaped area of the vestibule and inner labial fold is excised, followed by advancement of the posterior vaginal wall, has a better success rate.[8]

Referral to secondary care

Ideally, secondary care should be a team comprised of a gynaecologist, dermatologist, specialist from genitourinary medicine, psychosexual therapist and clinical psychologist. This is indicated if:

- the woman responds poorly to treatment
- the diagnosis is uncertain
- any suspicion of neoplasm[9]
- confirmed inflammatory skin disease of which symptoms can not be controlled in primary care.

KEY POINTS

- Vulvodynia is a chronic pain syndrome, still poorly understood and highly distressing for the patient.
- It can affect all or parts of the vulva.
- Women of all ages, races and socio-economic class can suffer from vulvodynia.
- A diagnosis of vulvodynia can be made on history and examination and further investigations may not be necessary.
- There is a small increased risk of cancer of the vulva affecting about 4 in 100 women with lichen sclerosis.
- Complete resolution of symptoms is difficult to achieve.
- The aim and objective of treatment is to minimise the symptoms and help women to lead as normal a life as possible.
- Most vulval problems can be managed adequately within primary care.
- Always refer a patient with chronic vulval pain to a specialist vulval service if not clear about the diagnosis.

Useful websites

For patients – helplines

British Association of Dermatologists information leaflet on vulvodynia and vestibulodynia:

www.bad.org.uk/site/884/default.aspx

British Pain Society: www.britishpainsociety.org/patient_publications.htm

National Vulvodynia Association, US non-profit organisation that aims to improve the lives of women with vulvodynia; provides education, networking, support awareness and advocacy: www.nva.org

NHS Choices: www.nhs.uk

Vulval Pain Society: www.vulvalpainsociety.org

Worldwide Lichen Sclerosis Support: www.lichensclerosus.net

For GPs

British Society for the Study of Vulval Disease: www.bssvd.org

International Society for the Study of Vulvovaginal Disease: www.issvd.org

Neill SM, Lewis FM, Tatnall FM. British Association of Dermatologists guidelines for the management of lichen sclerosus, 2010: www.bad.org.uk/Portals/_Bad/Guidelines/Clinical%20Guidelines/Lichen%20Sclerosus%20Guidelines%202010.pdf

Royal College of Obstetricians and Gynaecologists. Vulval skin disorders, management (Green-top 58): www.rcog.org.uk/womens-health/clinical-guidance/management-vulval-skin-disorders-green-top-58

References

1 Lynch PJ, Moyal-Banacco M. ISSVD Terminology Committee on Vulvar Pain. Terminology and classification. Available at: www.vulvodynia.com.au/general-information/terminology-classification/ (accessed 16 April 2013).

2 Harlow BL, Stewart EG. A population based assessment of chronic unexplained vulvar pain: have we underestimated the prevalence of vulvodynia. *J Am Med Womens Assoc.* 2003; **58**: 82–8. www.ncbi.nlm.nih.gov/pubmed/12744420

3 Bergeron S, Binik YM, Khalife S, *et al*. Vulvar vestibulitis syndrome, reliability of diagnosis and evaluation of current diagnostic criteria. *Obstet Gynecol.* 2001; **98**(1): 45–51.

4 Nunns D, Mandal D, Byrne M, *et al*. Guidelines for the management of vulvodynia. *Br J Dermatol.* 2010; 162: 1180–5.

5 Sobel J, Wiesenfeld H, Martens M, *et al*. Maintenance fluconazole therapy for recurrent vulvovaginal candidiasis. *N Engl J Med.* 2004; **351**(9): 876–83.

6 Neill SM, Lewis FM, Tatnall FM, *et al*. British Association of Dermatologists. British Association of Dermatologists guidelines for the management of lichen sclerosus. *Br J Dermatol.* 2010; **163**(4): 672–82.

7 Weijmar SWC, Gianotten WL, van der Meijden WI, *et al*. Behavioural approach with or without surgical intervention to the vulvar vestibulitis syndrome: a prospective randomised and non-randomised study. *J Psychosom Obstet Gynecol.* 1996; **17**(3): 143–8.

8 Kehoe S, Leusley D. An evaluation of modified vestibulectomy in the treatment of vulvar vestibulitis: preliminary results. *Acta Obstet Gynecol Scand.* 1996; **75**(7): 676–7.

9 Royal College of Obstetricians and Gynaecologists. The management of vulval skin disorders; 2011. Available at: www.rcog.org/files/rcog-corp/GTG58Vulval22022011.pdf (accessed 8 December 2012).

8

Management of vaginal discharge in primary care*

Vaginal discharge is a common presentation in primary care settings. It is important to establish at the outset the patient's concerns and the cause of this common symptom.

Aetiology

Physiological discharge

Physiological (normal) vaginal discharge is white, thin or creamy. Normal vaginal fluid is formed by mucous, dead skin cells shed from the surface of the vagina and cervix, white blood cells, and many different normal bacteria in addition to other proteins and fluids. It is normal and healthy for women of reproductive age to have some degree of vaginal discharge. The amount of vaginal discharge varies from woman to woman and changes as the level of oestrogen and progesterone levels change. Factors which cause an increase in the volume of vaginal discharge include ovulation and sexual arousal. Pregnancy also causes an increase in physiological discharge.

The vagina is colonised with commensal bacteria (normal vaginal flora) and lactobacilli. Lactobacilli metabolise glycogen in the vaginal epithelium to produce lactic acid. Thus the vaginal environment is acidic with pH levels ≤4.5. The acidic environment protects the vagina and uterus from pathogens.

Vaginal discharge is abnormal in prepubertal children and might indi-

---

* This chapter is based on guidance contained in Faculty of Sexual & Reproductive Healthcare. *Management of Vaginal Discharge in Non-Genitourinary Medicine Settings*. London: FSRH; 2012. Material reproduced with the kind permission of the Faculty of Sexual & Reproductive Healthcare Clinical Guidance.

cate sexual abuse or poor hygiene, resulting in increased growth of faecal organisms.

Vaginal discharge decreases in postmenopausal women due to a lack of oestrogens.

Pathological discharge

Pathological discharge can have infective or non-infective causes.

Infective (non-sexually transmitted):

- *Candida*
- bacterial vaginosis.

Infective (sexually transmitted):

- *Neisseria gonorrhoeae*
- *Chlamydia trachomatis*
- *Trichomonas vaginalis*
- herpes simplex virus.

Non-infective:

- foreign bodies (e.g. retained tampons, condoms)
- cervical polyps and ectopy
- genital tract malignancy
- fistulae
- atrophic vaginitis
- allergic or irritant reactions
- vulval dermatitis.

Non-sexually transmitted infections

Vulvovaginal candidiasis (VVC)

VVC is common among women of reproductive age. It is most commonly caused by *Candida albicans*. The *Candida* species of fungus is found naturally in the vagina, and is usually harmless. However, if conditions in the vagina change, *Candida albicans* may cause the symptoms of thrush. Symptoms of thrush can also be caused by *Candida glabrata, Candida krusei, Candida parapsilosis* and *Candida tropicalis*. Non-albican *Candida* is commonly found in complicated cases of vaginal thrush and is more likely in immunocompromised patients. Vaginal thrush is triggered by hormone imbalance due to antibiotics. VVC does not appear to be associated with tampons, sanitary towels or panty liners when they are used appropriately. As VVC can be found in non-sexually active individuals, it is not classed as an STI.

Bacterial vaginosis (BV)

BV is the most common cause of abnormal vaginal discharge in women of childbearing age, but may also be encountered in menopausal women. It is rare in children. Its prevalence in Caucasian women is 5%–15%, and in women of African origin it is 45%–55%. Its prevalence for Asian women is less well studied, but is estimated at around 20%–30%. It can occur and remit spontaneously and is characterised by an overgrowth of predominantly anaerobic organisms (e.g. *Gardnerella vaginalis*, *Prevotella* spp., *Mycoplasma hominis*, *Mobiluncus* spp.).[1] Typical signs and symptoms are shown in Table 8.1. BV is considered to be 'sexually associated' rather than truly 'sexually transmitted'. There is some evidence that consistent condom use may help to reduce BV prevalence.[2]

Factors increasing the risk of BV:

- douching
- intrauterine devices
- multiple sexual partners
- soap or shower gel
- menstruation.

Sexually transmitted infections

Neisseria gonorrhoeae

Gonorrhoea is caused by *Neisseria gonorrhoeae* and 50% of women are asymptomatic. It can present with increased or altered vaginal discharge and lower abdominal pain. Due to cervicitis it may present with postcoital or intermenstrual bleeding.[3]

Chlamydia trachomatis

Chlamydia trachomatis, the most common bacterial STI in the UK, is asymptomatic in approximately 70% of women. However, patients may present with purulent vaginal discharge due to cervicitis, abnormal bleeding (postcoital or intermenstrual) due to cervicitis, lower abdominal pain, dyspareunia or dysuria.[4]

Trichomonas vaginalis (TV)

TV is a flagellated protozoan that causes vaginitis. Women with TV commonly complain of vaginal discharge and dysuria. Typical signs and symptoms are shown in Table 8.1. TV is always sexually transmitted and is a rarer condition than BV or VVC.[5]

Herpes simplex

Women with cervicitis due to herpes simplex virus infection may occasionally present with vaginal discharge.

Other causes of vaginal discharge

Rarely vaginal discharge is due to foreign bodies (e.g. retained tampons or condoms), cervical ectopy or polyps, genital tract malignancy, fistulae, atrophic vaginitis, vulval dermatosis, allergic and irritant reactions. There is some association between methods of contraception and vaginal discharge. Women complaining of vaginal discharge should be asked about current and past contraception.

Women with cervical ectopy often complain of increased physiological discharge. These patients should be referred to secondary care. Silver nitrate cauterisation, laser or cold coagulation is the treatment of choice. Sinister cervical pathology must be excluded prior to treatment, and patients should be informed of potential risks and the fact that discharge symptoms may initially worsen before there is any improvement.

Primary care management

History

A proper history can distinguish between a physiological or pathological discharge. Enquire about:

- characteristics of discharge – onset, duration, colour and odour
- any cyclical variation in the amount and consistency of discharge
- any precipitating factors – sexual intercourse
- any associated symptoms – itching, urinary or bowel symptoms, abdominal pain/discomfort, abnormal bleeding
- menstrual history and any variation in volume or consistency of discharge
- reproductive history – pregnancy, postpartum or post abortion/termination
- contraceptive and sexual history
- any co-existing medical conditions – immuno-compromised state or diabetes mellitus
- past or present history of medications – antibiotics, contraceptive pills, corticosteroids.

Examination

The examination should include:

- inspection of the vulva (for obvious discharge, ulcers, other lesions or changes)
- speculum examination (colour of discharge, inspection of vaginal walls, cervix and foreign bodies).

Where there is any suggestion of upper genital tract infection, examination should also include:
- abdominal palpation (for tenderness/mass)
- bimanual pelvic examination (adnexal and/or uterine tenderness/mass, cervical motion tenderness).

TABLE 8.1 Symptoms and signs of infective causes of vaginal discharge

SYMPTOM/ SIGN	BACTERIAL VAGINOSIS *50% ASYMPTOMATIC*	CANDIDA *10%–20% ASYMPTOMATIC*	TRICHOMONIASIS *10%–50% ASYMPTOMATIC*
Discharge	Thin	Thick white, curdy	Scanty to profuse
Odour	Offensive/fishy	Non-offensive	Offensive
Itch	None	Vulval itch	Vulval itch
Other possible symptoms		Soreness Superficial dyspareunia Dysuria	Lower abdominal discomfort Dysuria
Visible signs	Discharge coating the vagina and vestibule No vulval inflammation	Vulval oedema Fissuring Satellite lesions	Frothy and yellow discharge (10%–30%) Vaginitis Strawberry cervix (2%)
Vaginal pH	>4.5	≤4.5	>4.5

Indications for referral to genitourinary medicine or a sexual health clinic include:
- gonorrhoea contact or positive nucleic acid amplification test (NAAT)
- suspected *Trichomonas* infection
- treatment failure, recurrent symptoms or diagnostic uncertainty
- pelvic inflammatory disease suspected
- blood-stained discharge.

Investigations
Ideally, all women presenting with vaginal discharge should be tested. If this is not possible, examination and testing must be performed if: TV detected on cervical cytology or diagnosed in a sexual partner; failure of vaginal discharge to respond to empirical treatment; severe or recurrent symptoms.[1]

Asymptomatic women do not require testing for BV or *Candida*.

A self-taken vulvovaginal swab (VVS) for chlamydia +/– gonorrhoea testing by NAAT is an option for patients declining examination.

Women appear to be very aware of VVC but less aware of BV, and it may be the case that women who self-diagnose with VVC may actually have other conditions.
- High vaginal swab (HVS): HVS is of limited value for diagnosing causes

of vaginal discharge. HVS may be used to diagnose of BV, VVC, TV or other genital tract infections (e.g. streptococcal organisms) but its use should generally be reserved for failed treatment and recurrent symptoms.

- If TV is suspected, referral to genitourinary medicine (GUM) is recommended for confirmation by wet microscopy +/− culture, and also for partner notification.
- Nucleic acid amplification test (NAAT): Combined chlamydia and gonorrhoea NAAT tests are now available and can be carried out on vulvovaginal, endocervix or urine samples. False-positives can occur with NAATs.

If gonorrhoea is suspected, an additional endocervical swab should be taken for microscopy, culture and sensitivity. Facilities for direct plating of samples for *N. gonorrhoeae* culture are not usually available in primary care, but transport medium (e.g. charcoal swab) gives acceptable results if plated immediately in the laboratory. If sending swabs to the laboratory in transport medium they should be stored at 4°C as soon as possible and transported to the laboratory ideally within 48 hours. Avoid fluctuations in temperature during transit.[3]

A culture should be taken in all cases of gonorrhoea diagnosed by NAATs prior to antibiotics being given, if possible, so that susceptibility testing can be performed and resistant strains identified.[3] A test of cure is also needed and should be referred to a local GUM clinic for partner notification.

Treatment
Treatment of non-sexually transmitted infections
Most cases of vaginal discharge can be treated in primary care. Advice about close fitting clothing, vaginal deodorants, bubble baths and vaginal douches must be given.

Bacterial vaginosis
Patients are advised to avoid vaginal douching, use of shower gel, and use of antiseptic agents or shampoos in the bath. Treatment is indicated for symptomatic women and women undergoing surgical procedures. The recommended treatments are metronidazole 400 mg twice daily for 5–7 days or intravaginal clindamycin cream (2%) once daily for 7 days. The alternative regimens are tinidazole 2 g single doses or clindamycin 300 mg twice daily for 7 days. All these treatments achieve cure rates of 70%–80% after 4 weeks.[2]

Non-antibiotic based treatment with probiotic lactobacilli or lactic acid preparations are not recommended at present. With metronidazole treatment, alcohol should be avoided because of the possibility of a disulfiram-like action. Both oral clindamycin and clindamycin cream can cause pseudo-membranous colitis.

Routine testing and treatment of male sexual partners is not currently recommended.

Vulvovaginal candidiasis
Vaginal and oral azole antifungals are equally effective in the treatment of VVC. There is no need for routine screening or treatment of sexual partners in the management of candidiasis.

Treatment of sexually transmitted infections
Trichomonas vaginalis
In the UK, first-line recommended treatment is oral metronidazole. As TV is an STI, treatment of partners is recommended. Test of cure is only recommended if symptoms persist or recur.

TABLE 8.2 Recommended treatment regimens

CONDITION	RECOMMENDED REGIMEN	ALTERNATIVE REGIMEN/ADVICE
BV	*Metronidazole 400 mg twice daily for 5–7 days, or 2 gm as a single dose; alternatively intravaginal metronidazole gel 0.75% can be used once a day for 5 days.	Intravaginal clindamycin cream (2%) once daily for 7 days or clindamycin** 300 mg capsule twice daily for 7 days or tinidazole tablet 2 g single dose Products that alter vaginal pH, such as gels containing lactic acid and glycogen, may be used as an alternative to drug treatment.
VVC	**Oral** Fluconazole 150 mg stat dose Itraconazole 200 mg bd for 1 day **Vaginal** Clotrimazole 500 mg pessary stat	If persistent or recurrent VVC refer to sexual health clinic
TV	**Oral** Metronidazole: single 2 g oral dose or 400 mg twice daily for 5–7 days	Tinidazole 2 g orally in a single dose
Chlamydia	Azithromycin 1 gm stat	Doxycycline 100 mg twice daily for 7 days
Gonorrhoea	Ceftriaxone 500 mg intramuscularly plus azithromycin 1 gm	Cefixime 400 mg stat if declined injection or as suggested by GC culture sensitivity

* There is no evidence of teratogenicity from use of metronidazole in the first trimester of pregnancy. Metronidazole is excreted in breast milk, so high doses should be avoided. Metronidazole can produce a disulfiram-like effect when taken with alcohol.

** Small amount of clindamycin can enter breast milk so intravaginal treatment is preferable. Intravaginal clindamycin can weaken condom.

Chlamydia and gonorrhoea

For the management of *Chlamydia* and gonorrhoea, refer to Table 8.2.

Management of vaginal discharge in special circumstances

Vaginal discharge in pregnancy

A woman's obstetrician should be informed of vaginal discharge symptoms in pregnancy and any tests or treatment given in primary care.

Bacterial vaginosis

In the UK, routine screening for BV in pregnant women is not currently recommended, but if BV is identified as a cause of vaginal discharge or as an incidental finding it should be treated.[2] Symptomatic pregnant women should be treated in the usual way. There is insufficient evidence to recommend routine treatment of asymptomatic pregnant women. Women with additional risk factors for preterm birth may benefit from treatment before 20 weeks' gestation. Although current evidence suggests that metronidazole is safe in pregnancy and is not teratogenic, single stat doses of 2 gm should be avoided.

Vulvovaginal candidiasis

VVC is common during pregnancy. There is no evidence of any adverse effect on pregnancy. Topical imidazoles (e.g. clotrimazole, econazole, miconazole) have been found to be effective in pregnant women with VVC but a longer treatment regimen may be required.[6] Oral antifungals should be avoided during pregnancy because of a lack of evidence of teratogenicity.

Women with VVC in pregnancy should avoid oral antifungals. Single-dose treatment is less effective than longer regimens of up to 7 days.

Trichomonas vaginalis

TV may be associated with preterm delivery and low birth weight. Over 90% of women are cleared of vaginal TV after treatment with metronidazole. Single stat dose of 2 gm metronidazole should be avoided. Current sexual partners of women diagnosed with TV should be offered a full sexual health screen and should be treated for TV irrespective of the results of their tests.

Recurrent vaginal discharge

If symptoms recur, referral to a specialist clinic (e.g. GUM, sexual health or vulval clinic) should be considered.

Recurrent BV

There is no specifically agreed definition of recurrent BV. Despite high initial cure rates, recurrence of BV is high. There are risk factors identified for recurrence and these include female, new or multiple sexual partners, oral sex, and copper-bearing intrauterine device (Cu-IUD) use. Most patients will have recurrences within 3–12 months, whatever treatment has been used. There is currently insufficient evidence to recommend the use of probiotics either before, during or after antibiotic treatment as a means of reducing recurrence.[2,7]

Recurrent VVC

Recurrent VVC is defined as four or more symptomatic mycological proven episodes per year.[1] After excluding risk factors (e.g. diabetes, underlying immunodeficiency, corticosteroid use, and frequent antibiotic use), consider for an initial intensive regimen of 10–14 days followed by a maintenance regimen, probably weekly for 6 months. Ovulation suppressing progesterone contraception (e.g. Depo-Provera or Cerazette) may have some benefits.

Recurrent TV

Recurrent TV is usually due to re-infection, although resistance to treatment can also be a cause. Treatment, advice on avoidance of sex or use of condoms and partner notification are required.

KEY POINTS

- The most common cause of increased vaginal discharge is physiological, BV and *Candida*, but STIs and non-infective causes must be considered and excluded.
- Self-taken vaginal NAAT tests for *Chlamydia* and gonorrhoea are available for use.
- Women appear to be very aware of VVC but less aware of BV, and therefore it may be that women who self-diagnose with VVC may actually have other conditions.
- During pregnancy, oral antifungals should be avoided.
- Pregnant or breastfeeding women with BV may use metronidazole 400 mg twice daily for 5–7 days. A 2 g stat dose of metronidazole is not recommended in pregnancy or breastfeeding women.

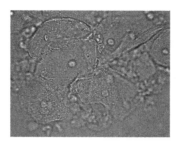

FIGURE 8.1 Wet mount – Normal vaginal epithelial cells

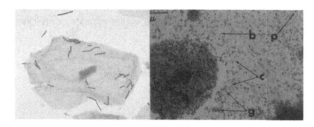

FIGURE 8.2 Gram-stained vaginal cell (normal vs BV)
Left: Normal vaginal epithelial cell with LB
Right: b – bacteroids; c – mobiluncus; g – gardnerella; p – peptostreptococci

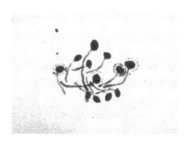

FIGURE 8.3 Vaginal smear gram stain: hyphae and spores

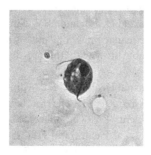

FIGURE 8.4 *Trichomonas vaginalis*

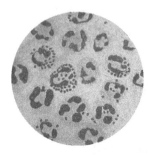

FIGURE 8.5 Cervical smear gram stain: intracellular diplococci (Gonococci)

Useful websites
For patients – helplines
www.patient.co.uk
www.nhs.uk

For GPs
www.bashh.org/guidelines
www.ffprhc.org.uk

References
1 Sherrard J, Donders G, White D. European (IUSTI/WHO) guideline on the management of vaginal discharge. *Int J STD AIDS.* 2011; **22**(8): 421–9.
2 British Association for Sexual Health and HIV Clinical Effectiveness Group. National guideline for the management of bacterial vaginosis. 2006. Available at: www.bashh.org/documents/62/62.pdf (accessed 2 August 2012).
3 British Association for Sexual Health and HIV Clinical Effectiveness Group. UK national guideline for the management of gonorrhoea in adults. 2012. Available at: www.bashh.org/documents/3611 (accessed 2 August 2012).
4 British Association for Sexual Health and HIV Clinical Effectiveness Group. UK national guideline for the management of genital tract infection with *Chlamydia trachomatis.* 2006. Available at: www.bashh.org/documents/0706.pdf (accessed 5 April 2013).
5 British Association for Sexual Health and HIV Clinical Effectiveness Group. UK national guideline on the management of *Trichomonas vaginalis.* 2007. Available at: www.bashh.org/documents/87/87.pdf (accessed 2 August 2012).
6 British Association of Sexual Health and HIV Clinical Effectiveness Group. Management of vulvovaginal candidiasis. 2007. Available at: www.bashh.org/documents/1798 (accessed 2 August 2012).

7 Centers for Disease Control and Prevention. Sexually transmitted diseases treatment guidelines. 2010. Available at: www.cdc.gov/std/treatment/2010/toc.htm (accessed 2 August 2012).

9

Pelvic inflammatory disease

DEFINITION

Pelvic inflammatory disease (PID) is an infection of the upper genital tract as a result of ascending infection from the endocervix causing endometritis, salpingitis, oophoritis, tubo-ovarian abscess and/or peritonitis.[1] It is one of the common GP gynaecological presentations and may range from clinical, subclinical to life-threatening disease.

Prevalence

In the UK, PID accounts for 1 in 60 GP consultations in female patients under the age of 45 years.[2] All sexually active women are at risk of developing PID. The incidence has risen over the past few years, resulting in an enormous impact on women's physical, mental and reproductive health.

Risk factors

Risk factors for PID include:
- multiple sexual partners[3]
- sexual intercourse at an early age[3]
- unprotected sexual intercourse
- previous pelvic infections
- young age (14–25 years) especially early age of first sexual intercourse
- lower socio-economic status
- vaginal douching
- instrumentation of uterus and or cervix
- coil insertion intrauterine device/intrauterine system (IUD/IUS) – relative risk is 1 in 1000.[3]

Aetiology

A majority of PIDs are associated with sexually transmitted infections:[4,5]
- *Chlamydia trachomatis* and *Neisseria gonorrhoea* are responsible for most cases of PID
- *Trichomonas vaginalis*
- *Gardnerella vaginalis*
- *Mycoplasma hominis*
- *Escherichia coli* (E. coli)
- *Actinomyces*
- *Mycobacterium tuberculosis* (TB)
- HIV.[1] Women with HIV infections have an increased risk of tubo-ovarian abscess formation.

Primary care management

Women with pelvic inflammatory disease may be completely asymptomatic and a diagnosis is made retrospectively upon presentation with primary or secondary infertility.

Acute cases present with:
- severe lower abdominal pain
- nausea and vomiting
- abnormal uterine bleeding – postcoital, menorrhagia or intermenstrual
- abnormal vaginal or cervical discharge
- dyspareunia
- perihepatitis in 10%–20%.

Chronic PID presents with:
- infertility
- recurrent pain of the lower abdomen – mild/moderate
- backache
- vaginal discharge
- abnormal vaginal bleeding
- dyspareunia.

Examination

General physical examination:
- temperature >38 degrees
- tachycardia
- hypotension
- pallor in acute cases.

Abdominal examination:
- bilateral lower abdominal tenderness
- rebound tenderness/guarding may be present
- tenderness in right upper quadrant may suggest Fitz-Hugh–Curtis syndrome.

Pelvic examination:
- tenderness in either fornix
- cervical excitation, cervicitis
- in some cases palpable adnexal mass
- muco-purulent discharge on per speculum examination.

Clinical signs and symptoms lack specificity and sensitivity with a predictive value of 65%–90%.[6]

Investigations
- Full blood count – high white cell count (WBC).
- Raised C-reactive protein (CRP).[7]
- Raised ESR.[7]
- Pregnancy test if pregnancy suspected.
- Liver function tests if suspected Fitz-Hugh–Curtis syndrome.
- Urinalysis for leucocytes and nitrite and if positive send for mid-stream urine for culture and sensitivity (MSU).
- High vaginal swab (HVS) to exclude bacterial vaginosis and trichomonal vaginalis.
- Endocervical swab for chlamydia and gonococcal infection.

A negative swab does not rule out a diagnosis of PID.[8]

Further investigations
- Pelvic ultrasound transvaginal examination if suspected tubo-ovarian abscess. There is insufficient evidence to support its use routinely.[9]
- Magnetic resonance imaging (MRI):[10] MRI is recommended over computerised tomography (CT) because there is no risk of radiation and it is 93% sensitive.
- CT scan.[11]
- Laparoscopy: if in doubt, a laparoscopy can exclude other pathologies.[12] Routine laparoscopy is not advised because of its 15%–30% likelihood of a false negative result.[13]

Differential diagnosis
- Acute appendicitis.

- Endometriosis.
- Ectopic pregnancy.
- Irritable bowel syndrome (IBS).
- Rupture or torsion of ovary.
- Urinary tract infection (UTI).

Prevention

Pelvic inflammatory disease may be prevented by:

- using barrier methods – durex or caps/diaphragms
- early diagnosis and early treatment of urethritis or cystitis
- routine screening of sexually transmitted infections (STIs) in high-risk patients
- nutrition, supplements and herbs. There is no firm medical evidence, however simple health promotional advice regarding increasing fluid intake, cutting down on alcohol and caffeine and stopping smoking should be offered.

Admission to hospital

Admit patient to hospital in the following scenarios:

- temperature of 38 degrees or more
- vomiting, tachycardia, dehydration
- suspected ectopic pregnancy
- suspected acute appendicitis
- suspected tubo-ovarian abscess or pelvic mass
- pelvic inflammatory disease in pregnancy
- patient suffering from immunodeficiency
- diagnosis uncertainty.

Treatment

The patient will require:

- rest
- adequate analgesia
- an early treatment with broad spectrum antibiotic to avoid long-term tubal damage and risk of future ectopic pregnancy.

All patients suspected of PID should be referred to secondary care. Most primary care practices operate on a 'choose and book' system for referral. A decision as to whether the patient can be seen as an outpatient or needs admission depends on the clinical condition of the patient.

Outpatient treatment can be as effective as inpatient treatment for mild cases of PID, but if in doubt: ADMIT.

Treatment regime

The decision to treat as inpatient or outpatient should be initiated by the consultant. Recommended regimens are based on the RCOG 2008 update.[1]

Outpatient antibiotics treatment

Oral ofloxacin 400 mg twice daily plus oral metronidazole 400 mg twice daily for 14 days, intramuscular ceftriaxone 250 mg single dose followed by doxycycline 100 mg twice daily plus metronidazole 400 mg twice daily for 14 days.[14,15] Metronidazole may be discontinued in women who are unable to tolerate it.

Inpatient antibiotics treatment

Ofloxacin 400 mg orally 12 hourly or doxycycline 100 mg orally 12 hourly. Ofloxacin should be avoided if gonococcal pelvic inflammatory disease is suspected.

AND Metronidazole 400 mg orally 12 hourly. Oral therapy should be for 14 days.

OR

Ceftriaxone 2 gm by intravenous infusion daily plus intravenous doxycycline 100 mg twice daily, followed by oral doxycycline 100 mg twice daily plus oral metronidazole 400 mg twice daily for 14 days.[14,15]

OR

Intravenous clindamycin 900 mg three times daily plus intravenous gentamicin followed by either oral clindamycin 450 mg four times daily for 14 days OR oral doxycycline 100 mg twice daily plus oral metronidazole 400 mg twice daily for 14 days.[15]

OR

Intravenous ofloxacin 400 mg twice daily plus intravenous metronidazole 500 mg three times daily for 14 days.[14,15]

All intravenous treatment is continued until 24 hours after clinical improvement. Patients can be switched to oral treatment if clinically appropriate. Treatment must be continued even in the absence of positive swab results.

Management of women with an intrauterine contraceptive device

If an IUD is in situ, and this is the preferred method of contraception, it should be left in place. Removal of an IUD should be considered in women with PID, especially in those whose symptoms do not settle within 72 hours and other causes of pain have been excluded.[16,17] The risk of unsuspected pregnancy must be assessed carefully if there is a clear history of unprotected sexual intercourse in the preceding 7 days. The patient must be involved in the decision making and given a hormonal postcoital pill.

Pelvic inflammatory disease and pregnancy

All women must have a pregnancy test to exclude ectopic pregnancy. Pelvic inflammatory disease is rare with intrauterine pregnancy except in cases of septic abortion. Pregnant women with confirmed chlamydia and gonococcal infection must be treated with a combination of ceftriaxone, azithromycin and metronidazole for 14 days. Tetracyclines should be avoided in pregnancy because of toxicity.

Management of sexual partners

If a sexually transmitted infection is found to be the cause of pelvic inflammatory disease, the current sexual partner/partners should be screened and treated.[1]

Women with HIV

Women with HIV may experience more severe pelvic inflammatory disease but should be treated with the same antibiotic regimes as women who are HIV negative. They should be referred to an HIV physician.[18]

Follow up appointment

All patients should be seen at 4–6 weeks to:
- ensure good clinical response
- ensure compliance with treatment
- receive advice regarding prevention of future episodes and seek help promptly if the symptoms return
- seek contraceptive advice
- repeat pregnancy test if indicated
- carry out screening and treatment of sexual partners; one study of women with acute salpingitis found that 30 out of 34 male contacts had urethritis.[19]

Sequelae

Even a few days of delay regarding appropriate treatment increases the risk of the following sequelae:[20]

- subfertility in 20%[21]
- chronic pelvic pain in 20%[21]
- Ten per cent of those who conceive have an ectopic pregnancy[21]
- tubo-ovarian abscesses
- permanent tubal damage with repeated episodes of PID[22]
- rarely Fitz-Hugh–Curtis syndrome; infection resulting in perihepatic adhesions due to spread of infection to the liver capsule.

KEY POINTS

- PID is a common cause of morbidity and accounts for 1 in 60 GP consultations of women under 45 years of age.[1]
- PID may be asymptomatic.
- It is likely that delaying treatment increases the risk of long-term sequelae such as ectopic pregnancy, infertility and pain.
- A more severe disease can result in adverse sequelae which can result in significant healthcare costs.[23]
- Because of the lack of definitive diagnostic criteria, a low threshold for empiric treatment is recommended.
- Clear documentation in the consultation notes is important to avoid medico-legal implications.

Useful websites

For patients – helplines

Ectopic pregnancy Trust: www.ectopic.org.uk

Pelvic Pain Support Network: www.pelvicpain.org.uk

Royal College of Obstetricians and Gynaecologists patient leaflets on acute pelvic inflammatory disease, ectopic pregnancy, bleeding and pain in early pregnancy, miscarriage: www.rcog.org.uk/women-health/patient-information

'Women's health' and 'pelvic inflammatory disease' in www.patient.co.uk

For GPs

Bacterial vaginosis: Bacterial Vaginosis BASHH. www.bash.org/documents/62/62.pdf. National Guideline For The Management of Bacterial Vaginosis (2006) Clinical Effectiveness Group. British Association For Sexual Health And HIV.

Candida: National Guideline on the Management of Vulvovaginal Candidiasis www.bashh.org/documents/50/50.pdf

Pelvic inflammatory disease, NHS: www.nhs.uk/conditions/pelvic-inflammatory-disease

The Association of Early Pregnancy Units: www.earlypregnancy.org.uk

References

1 Royal College of Obstetricians and Gynaecologists (RCOG). Pelvic inflammatory disease. Green-top guideline 32. 17 November 2008. Available at: www.rcog.org.uk/womens-health/clinical-guidance/management-acute-pelvic-inflammatory-disease-32 (accessed 13 December 2012).

2 Simms I, Vickers MR, Stephenson J, *et al*. National assessment of PID diagnosis, treatment and management in general practice: England and Wales. *Int J STD AIDS*. 2000; **11**(7): 440–4.

3 Crossman SH. The challenge of pelvic inflammatory disease. *Am Fam Physician*. 2006; **73**(5): 859–64. Available at: www.umm-edu/altmed/articles/pelvic-inflam-000124.htm (accessed 13 December 2012).

4 Simms I, Eastick K, Mallinson H, *et al*. Associations between *Mycoplasma genitalium*, *Chlamydia trachomatis*, and pelvic inflammatory disease. *Sex Transm Infect*. 2003; **79**(2): 154–6.

5 Baveja G, Saini S, Sangwan K, *et al*. A study of bacterial pathogens in acute pelvic inflammatory disease. *J Commun Dis*. 2001; **33**(2): 121–5.

6 Gaitan H, Angel E, Diaz R, *et al*. Accuracy of five different diagnostic techniques in mild to moderate pelvic inflammatory disease. *Infec Dis Obstet Gynecol*. 2002; **10**(4): 171–80.

7 Miettinen AK, Heinonen PK, Laippala P, *et al*. Test performance of erythrocyte sedimentation rate and C-reactive protein in assessing the severity of acute pelvic inflammatory disease. *Am J Obstet Gynecol*. 1993; **169**(5): 1143–9.

8 Ross JDC. An update on pelvic inflammatory disease. *Sex Transm Infect*. 2002; **78**(1): 18–19.

9 Taipale P, Tarjanne H, Ylostalo P. Transvaginal sonography in suspected pelvic inflammatory disease. *Ultrasound Obstet Gynecol*. 1995; **6**(6): 430–4.

10 Bennett GL, Slywotzky CM, Glovanniello G. Gynecologic causes of acute pelvic pain: spectrum of CT findings. *Radiographics*. 2002; **22**(4): 785–801.

11 Tukeva TA, Aronen HJ, Karjalainen PT, *et al*. MR imaging in pelvic inflammatory disease: comparison with laparoscopy and US. *Radiology*. 1999; 201: 209–16.

12 Cibula D, Kuzel D, Fucikova Z, *et al*. Acute exacerbation of recurrent pelvic inflammatory disease. Laparoscopic findings in 141 women with a clinical diagnosis. *J Reprod Med*. 2001; **46**(1): 49–53.

13 Morcos R, Frost N, Hnat M, *et al*. Laparoscopic versus clinical diagnosis of acute pelvic inflammatory disease. *J Reprod Med*. 1993; **38**(1): 53–6.

14 Martens MG, Gordon S, Yarborough DR, *et al*. Multicenter randomized trial of ofloxacin versus cefoxitin and doxycycline in outpatient treatment of pelvic inflammatory disease. Ambulatory PID Research Group. *Southern Med J*. 1993; **86**(6): 604–10.

15 Walker CK, Kahn JG, Washington AF, *et al*. Pelvic inflammatory disease: meta-analysis of antimicrobial regime efficacy. *J Infect Dis*. 1993; **168**(4): 969–78.

16 Teisala K. Removal of an IUD and the treatment of acute PID. *Annals of Medicine*. 1989; 21: 63–5.

17 Soderberg G, Lingren S. Influence of an IUD on the course of acute salpingitis. *Contraception*. 1981; 24: 137–43.

18 Irwin KL, Moorman AC, O'Sullivan MJ, *et al*. Influence of human immunodeficiency virus infection on pelvic inflammatory disease. *Obstet Gynaecol*. 2000; **95**(4): 525–34.

19 Kinghorn GR, Duerden BI, Hafiz S. Clinical and microbiological investigation of women with acute salpingitis and their consorts. *Br J Obstet Gynaecol*. 1986; **93**(8): 869–80.

20 Hillis SD, Joesoef R, Marchbanks PA, *et al*. Delayed care of pelvic inflammatory disease as a risk factor for impaired fertility. *Am J Obstet Gynacol*. 1993; **168**(5): 1503–9.

21 Metters JS, Catchpole M, Smith C, *et al*. Chlamydia trachomatis: summary and conclusions of CMO's expert advisory group. London: Department of Health; 1998.

22 Hills SD, Owens LM, Marchbanks PA, *et al*. Recurrent chlamydial infections increase the risks of hospitalisation for ectopic pregnancy and pelvic inflammatory disease. *Am J Obstet Gynecol*. 1997; 176: 103–7.

23 Yeh JM, Hook EW 3rd, Goldie SJ. A refined estimate of the average lifetime cost of pelvic inflammatory disease. *Sex Transm Dis*. 2003; **30**(5): 369–8.

10

Dysfunctional uterine bleeding

DEFINITION

Dysfunctional uterine bleeding (DUB) is defined as abnormal uterine bleeding in the absence of organic disease[1]. It usually presents as menorrhagia and affects women's health both medically and socially. Menorrhagia is defined as a blood loss greater than 80 ml. An irregular and prolonged period is called metrorrhagia.

Dysfunctional uterine bleeding is therefore a diagnosis of exclusion and can only be made once all other causes for abnormal or heavy uterine bleeding have been excluded.

Prevalence

DUB is more common in adolescents and perimenopausal women, as most cases are associated with anovulatory menstrual cycles. Among women aged 30–49 years, 1 in 20 consults her general practitioner each year with menorrhagia,[1] making dysfunctional uterine bleeding one of the most often encountered gynaecological problems.

Heavy menstrual loss accounts for 12% of all gynaecological referrals in the UK.[2] About 30% of all women complain of menorrhagia, and it accounts for two thirds of all hysterectomies and most endoscopic endometrial destructive surgery.[3] Only 2% of endometrial carcinomas occur before the age of 40. Each year around £7 million is spent in the UK on prescriptions in primary care to treat menorrhagia.[1]

Aetiology[4]

DUB reflects a disruption in the normal cyclic pattern of endometrial stimulation that arises from an ovulatory cycle. As a result there are constant, noncycling oestrogen levels that stimulate endometrial growth. This endometrium continues to proliferate without periodic shedding, causing the endometrium to outgrow its blood supply. Eventually, this out-of-phase endometrium is shed in an irregular and dyssynchronous manner. The bleeding becomes unpredictable and may be excessively heavy or light, prolonged, frequent or random. Ovulatory DUB occurs secondary to defects in the local endometrial haemostasis.[1]

Differential diagnosis

- Uterine pathology – fibroids, endometrial polyps or hyperplasia, carcinoma, endometriosis and infection. Endometrial hyperplasia is classified as simple, complex or atypical. Simple and complex hyperplasias carry a 1%–3% risk of malignant transformation and atypical hyperplasia carries a risk of 23%–29%.[12]
- Cervical pathology – cervicitis, cervical cancer.
- Systemic disease – hypo/hyperthyroidism, PCOS, obesity, hyperprolactaenemia, liver disease, haematological disorders (e.g. von Willebrand disease).
- Iatrogenic causes – intrauterine device, medication (e.g. HRT), oral contraceptives, anticoagulants.
- Pregnancy – ectopic, threatened or incomplete miscarriage.

Primary care management

History

- Menstrual history:
  — cycle length
  — duration of bleeding
  — degree of blood loss, i.e. number of pads/tampons changed per day, passage of clots, flooding and leakage
  — associated intermenstrual (IMB) or postcoital bleeding (PCB)
  — associated dysmenorrhoea.
- Contraception: current method, is family complete?
- Exclude pregnancy
- Symptoms suggesting underlying pathology:
  — metabolic disorders, e.g. PCOS, hypothyroidism
  — bleeding disorders, e.g. easy bruising, bleeding gums, epistaxis, excessive bleeding during dental procedures or childbirth

— pelvic inflammatory disease (PID) – pelvic pain, dyspareunia, vaginal discharge
— endometriosis – pelvic pain, dysmenorrhoea
— intermenstrual bleed (IMB) or postcoital bleed (PCB).

Examination

General physical examination:

- obesity (BMI)
- pallor
- bruising
- features of hypo/hyperthyroidism
- features of PCOS – hirsutism, acne, obesity
- galactorrhoea – may suggest hyperprolactinaemia.

Abdominal:

- lower abdominal tenderness
- palpable masses – uterine, ovarian.

Pelvic:

- vulval inspection
- speculum examination
- bimanual examination for masses
- cervical smear – if appropriate.

Investigations

The investigation should cover the following:

- full blood count in all women[5]
- coagulation screen in adolescents
- liver function test (LFT) – if alcoholism or hepatitis suspected; any condition affecting liver metabolism of oestrogen can be associated with abnormal uterine bleeding
- cervical smear – if appropriate
- infection screening – high vaginal swab (HVS) and endocervical swab (ECS) if appropriate
- serum ferritin, thyroid function test (TFT), follicle stimulating hormone (FSH) and luteinising hormone (LH) are not routinely recommended and should be carried out only if there is a strong clinical suspicion of underlying pathology.[5]

Further investigations

- Pelvic ultrasound scan: first line diagnostic tool for identifying structural abnormalities.

- Hysteroscopy and endometrial biopsy: 'one stop' hysteroscopy clinic in primary care with an ultrasound facility can make an early diagnosis and reduce the unnecessary referrals to secondary care. Any suspected cancer can be referred to secondary care under a 2-week rule.

Referral to secondary care
The patient should be referred to secondary care if:
- woman >45 years with heavy menstrual bleeding
- persistent menstrual bleeding
- abnormalities are detected on examination
- increased risk of pathology from history, e.g. null parity, tamoxifen, PCOS
- abnormal smear
- failure of medical treatment.

If a referral to specialist care is being made, the woman should be given information before her outpatient appointment.[5]

Medical management
The first-line management of DUB is pharmaceutical treatment once organic causes for heavy menstrual bleeding have been excluded. Iron supplements should be given to all anaemic patients.

Treatments should be considered in the following order:

First-line treatment
- **Levonorgestrel-releasing intrauterine system**, provided long-term use (at least 12 months) is anticipated.
- It prevents endometrial proliferation and also acts as a contraceptive.
- Equally as effective as hysterectomy in improving quality of life and psychological well-being.[6,7]
- Side effects include irregular bleeding lasting up to 6 months, progesterone-related problems (e.g. breast tenderness, acne, headaches, pelvic pain), rarely uterine perforation at insertion.

Second-line treatment
A Tranexamic acid *or*
B Non-steroidal anti-inflammatory drugs (NSAIDs) *or*
C The combined oral contraceptive pill (COCP).

A Tranexamic acid
- This is an oral antifibrinolytic.

- Treatment should be stopped if no improvement after 3 cycles.
- The usual dose is 1–1.5 g three to four times daily, taken for three to four days on the heaviest days of the cycle.
- Side effects include nausea, vomiting, diarrhoea and allergic skin reaction.
- There has been reluctance to prescribe it due to potential increased risk of thrombosis, but a Cochrane review has showed that there are no data available within randomised controlled trials that record the frequency of thromboembolic events during treatment with tranexamic acid.[8]

B NSAIDs
- These reduce the production of prostaglandin.
- Treatment should be stopped if no improvement after three cycles.
- The commonly used NSAID is mefenamic acid and this is preferred over tranexamic acid if associated dysmenorrhoea, although both can be used together.
- The usual dose is 500 mg three times a day during heavy bleeding.
- Side effects include dyspepsia, diarrhoea, headaches and worsening of asthma.

C COCPs
- Prevent proliferation of the endometrium.
- Also act as a contraceptive but do not impact future fertility.
- Side effects include mood swings, headache, nausea, fluid retention, thrombosis and cervical ectropion.

Tranexamic acid or NSAIDs can be used as first-line medical treatment if hormonal treatments are unacceptable to the woman.

Third-line treatment
A Norethisterone 15 mg daily from days 5–26 of the menstrual cycle *or*
B Injected long-acting progestogens (Depo-Provera).[5]

A Norethisterone
- Prevents proliferation of the endometrium.
- Also acts as a contraceptive but does not impact future fertility.
- The usual dose is 5 mg three times a day from days 5–26 of the cycle.
- Side effects include weight gain, bloating, breast tenderness, headaches and depression.
- A recent Cochrane review showed that cyclical progestogen therapy results in a significant reduction in menstrual blood loss, but the

women found the treatment less acceptable than intrauterine levonorgestrel.[9]

B Depo-Provera
- Prevents proliferation of the endometrium.
- Also acts as a contraceptive but does not impact future fertility.
- Side effects include weight gain, bloating, breast tenderness, fluid retention and bone density loss.
- Due to the potential for bone density loss, current guidance is that depot-medroxyprogesterone acetate should only be used in adolescents if other treatments for heavy menstrual bleeding are unsuitable, ineffective or unacceptable. In women of all ages, careful re-evaluation of the risks and benefits of use should be carried out at two years. If there are significant risk factors for osteoporosis, alternative treatment for heavy menstrual bleeding should be considered first.[10]

Arresting very heavy bleeding
In the acute situation of disabling bleeding, treatment with high-dose norethisterone (30 mg daily) can be used. This is continued until the bleeding is controlled, and then the dose is tailed off.

Surgical management
Consider only if:
- medical treatment has failed
- there is severe impact on quality of life
- there is no desire to conceive
- the uterus is normal (or there are just small fibroids <3 cm).

Options for surgical management
First-line
Endometrial ablation
- (Second generation): non-hysteroscopic; no general anaesthetic required; shorter recovery time.
- Bipolar radiofrequency ablation.
- Balloon thermal ablation.
- Microwave ablation.
- Free fluid thermal ablation.

or

- (First generation): hysteroscopic; general anaesthetic usually required.
- Rollerball ablation (a current is passed through a rollerball electrode that is moved around the endometrium).
- Transcervical resection of the endometrium (the endometrial lining ± small fibroids are removed using a cutting loop).

Unwanted outcomes of endometrial ablation:
- vaginal discharge
- increased period pain even if no further bleeding
- treatment failure and therefore require a repeat procedure or move on to hysterectomy
- infection
- perforation (very rare).

Contraception after endometrial ablation is still advised as some studies report up to 5% pregnancy rate in post-ablation procedures.[4]

Second-line

Hysterectomy
Consider only if:
- other treatments have failed, are contra-indicated or declined
- there is desire for amenorrhoea
- the woman is fully informed and requests it
- there is no desire to retain the uterus and fertility
- vaginal hysterectomy in preference to abdominal where possible
- healthy ovaries are conserved.

COST-EFFECTIVE TREATMENT

The authors of a recent study concluded that in light of the acceptable thresholds used by NICE, hysterectomy would be considered the preferred strategy for the treatment of heavy menstrual bleeding. The incremental cost-effectiveness ratio for hysterectomy compared with second generation ablation is £970 per additional quality adjusted life years (QALY) and compared with the LING-IUS is £1,440 per additional QALY.[11]

Recent developments
Recent developments include the use of bipolar resectoscope, which can 'see and treat' at the same time. The advantages are fewer days in hospital, faster recovery and early return to work.

Unwanted outcomes of hysterectomy:

- infection
- intraoperative haemorrhage
- damage to other organs, e.g. bladder, ureters and bowel
- urinary dysfunction
- thrombosis
- menopausal symptoms if ovaries are removed
- postoperative adhesions.

Sequelae

- Iron-deficiency anaemia.
- Social: cost of pads and tampons; time off work.
- Psychological: depression; embarrassment.
- Endometrial cancer: 1%–2% of women with improperly managed anovulatory bleeding eventually might develop endometrial cancer.[4]

KEY POINTS

- The hallmark of DUB is a negative examination despite the clinical history.
- Heavy but regular uterine bleeding implies ovular bleeding and should not be diagnosed as DUB.
- The goals of treatment are to stop the acute bleeding, avert future episodes and prevent long-term complications.
- Patients need to be educated that after the initial treatment and resolution, chronic therapy may be needed to prevent further episodes.

Useful websites

For patients – helplines

www.patient.co.uk
www.nice.org.uk/patientsandpublic

For GPs

Behera MA, Price TM, Queenan JT Jr. Clinical Fact Sheet. Abnormal Uterine Bleeding. Available at: www.arhp.org/publications-and.../abnormal-uterine-bleeding.

References

1 Pitkin J. Dysfunctional uterine bleeding. *BMJ*. 2007 May 26; **334**(7603): 1110–11.

2 Lethaby AE, Cooke I, Rees M. Progesterone or progestogen-releasing intrauterine systems for heavy menstrual bleeding. Cochrane Database Syst Rev. 2007; 2.

3 Oehler MK, Rees MC. Menorrhagia: an update. *Acta Obstet Gynecol Scand.* 2003 May; **82**(5): 405–22. [abstract]

4 Behera MA, Price TM. Dysfunctional uterine bleeding. e-Medicine. June 2009.

5 National Institute for Health and Clinical Excellence. Heavy Menstrual Bleeding: NICE guideline 54. London: NIHCE; 2007. www.nice.org.uk/CG44

6 Hurskainen R, Teperi J, Rissanen P, *et al.* Quality of life and cost-effectiveness of levonorgestrel-releasing intrauterine system versus hysterectomy for treatment of menorrhagia: a randomised trial. *Lancet.* 2001 Jan 27; **357**(9252): 273–7. [abstract]

7 Marjoribanks J, Lethaby A, Farquhar C. Surgery versus medical therapy for heavy menstrual bleeding. Cochrane Database Syst Rev. 2006; 2: CD003855. [abstract]

8 Lethaby A, Farquhar C, Cooke I. Antifibrinolytics for heavy menstrual bleeding. Cochrane Database Syst Rev. 2000; 4: CD000249. [abstract]

9 Lethaby A, Irvine G, Cameron I. Cyclical progestogens for heavy menstrual bleeding. Cochrane Database Syst Rev. 2008; 1: CD001016.

10 British National Formulary No. 63 (March 2012): www.medicinescomplete.com/mc/bnf/current

11 Roberts TE, Tsourapas A, Middleton LJ. Hysterectomy, endometrial ablation and levonorgestrel releasing intrauterine system (Mirena) for treatment of heavy menstrual bleeding: cost effectiveness analysis. *BMJ*. 2011; 342: d2202. Available at: www.ncbi.nlm.nih.gov/pubmed/21521730 (accessed 13 December 2012).

12 Kurman RJ, Kaminski PF, Norris HJ. The behaviour of endometrial hyperplasia. A long term study of untreated hyperplasia in 170 patients. *Cancer.* 1985; **56**(2); 403–12.

REFERRAL GUIDE: Menorrhagia

Clinical presentation

- Excessive menstrual blood loss that interferes with the patient's quality of life
- Nature and degree of blood loss, e.g. flooding, clots
- Age at menarche
- Cycle length including variability and duration of blood loss and heaviest days
- **Red flag symptoms:** persistent intermenstrual bleeding; postcoital bleeding; sudden increase in blood loss; persistent symptoms in a woman over 45 years despite treatment
- Assess associated symptoms, e.g. dysmenorrhoea, dyspareunia, pelvic pain and pressure symptoms

Examination

- Not absolutely necessary in the first instance if there are no symptoms suggesting an underlying cause and only oral therapy planned as first-line*
- Assess for systemic signs of disease, e.g. hirsutism, bruising. etc.
- Abdominal examination for masses arising from pelvis and organomegaly
- Pelvic examination: inspect vulva for possible local cause of bleeding, speculum examination of vagina and cervix and bi-manual examination to assess uterine size, regularity, adnexal masses or tenderness
- **Red flag signs:** pelvic mass that is not fibroids, vulval lump or vulval bleeding due to ulceration

Investigations

- Full blood count: treat iron deficiency anaemia with oral iron
- HVS and endocervical swabs if infection suspected
- Investigations for underlying condition if suspected
- Ultrasound scan if structural abnormality suspected from history or examination findings

Primary/community provision prior to specialist opinion (unless indication for early referral)

Therapy should be tried in the following order apart from when no examination has been performed as above*

1. Levonorgestrel-releasing intrauterine system (examination prior to insertion required)
2. Tranexamic acid, NSAID or combined oral contraceptive pill
3. Oral progestogen: norethisterone 5 mg three times a day for 3 weeks from day 5 of cycle
4. Injected progestogen: 150 mg medroxyprogesterone IM

Indication for referral for specialist opinion

- **Red flag symptoms and/or signs:** if cancer suspected use 2ww referral pathway
- Failure of at least two of the primary care treatment steps

11

Postmenopausal bleeding

DEFINITION

Postmenopausal bleeding (PMB) is defined as spontaneous vaginal bleeding than occurs 12 months or more after the last period, in a woman of menopausal age.[1]

Unscheduled bleeding, not PMB, is the term that should be used for breakthrough bleeding occurring in women on cyclical HRT or any bleeding in women on tibolone (Livial) or continuous combined HRT.

Prevalence

PMB is a common problem, representing 5% of all gynaecology outpatient attendances.[2] Endometrial cancer is present in approximately 10% of patients referred with PMB.[1] The risk of endometrial cancer in women on combined hormone replacement therapy (HRT) presenting with PMB or unscheduled bleeding is 1%,[1] while the risk for women on continuous combined HRT is assumed to be similar to those not on HRT.

Risk factors[3]

Risk factors may include:

- nulliparity
- obesity (often associated with diabetes and hypertension)
- history of chronic anovulation, e.g. polycystic ovarian syndrome (PCOS)
- exposure to unopposed oestrogen
- strong family history of endometrial or colon cancer (Lynch syndrome)
- exposure to tamoxifen (risk rises with duration of therapy and increasing dose)

- anticoagulants
- endometrial thickness >8 mm.

Aetiology

Contributing factors may include:
- use of hormone replacement therapy (HRT)
- vaginal atrophy
- endometrial hyperplasia: simple, complex and atypical
- endometrial carcinoma
- endometrial polyps or cervical polyps
- cervical carcinoma
- ring pessary
- ovarian carcinoma – oestrogen-secreting tumour
- vaginal carcinoma (very uncommon)
- vulval carcinoma
- non-gynaecological: trauma, bleeding disorder.

Primary care management

Any PMB should be assumed to be malignant, until proven otherwise. Therefore the principal aim of investigating PMB is to identify or exclude endometrial pathology, most notably endometrial carcinoma. This requires the patient to be seen by a gynaecologist within 2 weeks of referral.[4] In Oldham, GPs use the pro-forma template shown in Figure 11.1.

History
- Last day of menstrual period (LMP).
- Identification of risk factors.
- Pattern of bleeding:
  — how long and how heavy?
  — associated with intercourse?
  — previous episodes?
- Associated vaginal discharge:
  — dark-stained blood or 'unusual for the woman' discharge is a possible symptom of endometrial cancer.
- History of any associated pain:
  — smear history
  — drug history:
    ¤ On HRT? If so is there a problem that suggests poor compliance; poor gastrointestinal absorption (e.g. gastroenteritis); drug interactions; coagulation defects.

¤ on Tamoxifen?
- Functional enquiry – recent weight loss or loss of appetite?

The patient will usually be able to clarify where the bleeding is coming from. In case of any uncertainty, a tampon may be inserted in the vagina to confirm.

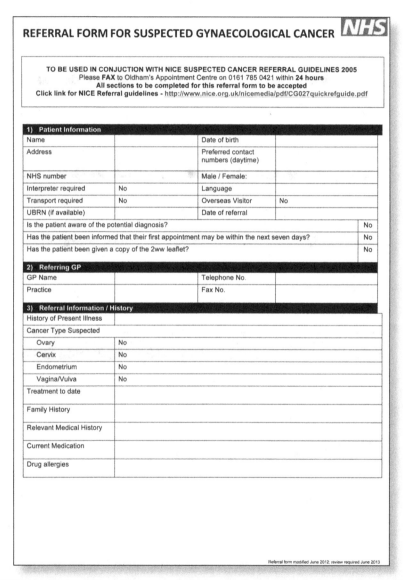

FIGURE 11.1 Referral form for suspected gynaecological cancer. Reproduced with permission

Examination

General examination

- Height, weight, BMI – any weight loss or weight gain?
- Blood pressure – documenting the blood pressure reading in the referral letter is not only courteous but will also benefit the patient.

Page 2

Surname:

NHS Number

4) Symptoms						
Bleeding PV:	Inter menstrual	No	Postcoital	No	Postmenopausal	No
Alterations in menstrual cycle		No	Indigestion			No
Vaginal discharge		No	Lower Back Pain			No
Bloating		No	Difficulty in passing urine and faeces			No
Abdominal swelling		No	Pain having sexual intercourse			No
Unexplained abdominal symptoms >1 or a single heavy episode of post menopausal bleed in women who are NOT on HRT						No
Unexpected or prolonged bleeding persisting for >4 weeks after stopping HRT						No

5) Clinical Examination	
Abdominal Mass	No
Palpable pelvic mass (not fibroids) or suspicious pelvic mass on ultrasound (not fibroids)	No
Lesion suspicious of cancer on cervix/vagina on speculum examination, or vulva on clinical examination	No
Other (please describe in detail the findings on your examination)	

6) Diagnostic Investigations / Results			
CA125 result (for suspected ovarian malignancy only)		Date	
NB: If CA125 result is not available, please request at the point of referral			
Transvaginal / abdominal ultrasound result		Date	
Last smear result		Date	

Mandatory Diagnostic Information

U&E sent at the time of the referral or within the last 3 months	No	eGFR result (if known)	

Without this information the patient pathway is delayed (CT cannot be undertaken without eGFR due to the risk of contrast nephropathy). Most 2ww referrals require staging CT.

7) Additional / Supporting Information / Patient Concerns

Receiving Clinician only	
Was this referral in line with referral criteria?	Yes / No If not, why not?
Action Taken	

Receiving clinician – please send a photocopy of this to the Cancer Services Offices

Referral form modified June 2012; review required June 2013

FIGURE 11.1 Referral form (cont.)

Abdominal examination

- It is good medical practice to examine the abdomen for any masses and check for an enlarged liver. Abdominal palpation may detect an enlarged uterus.

Pelvic examination

- All women should have a bimanual pelvic examination to determine the size, mobility and tenderness of the uterus and to exclude non-uterine pelvic masses.
- Examination should include inspection of the vulva to exclude vulval dystrophy or vulval carcinoma. Look for urethral caruncle. Check vagina to exclude vaginal atrophy or vaginal carcinoma. Per speculum examination must be done to exclude any suspicious looking lesion, erosion or polyp of the cervix.

Continuation of HRT prior to investigation[1]

- There is uncertainty as to whether HRT should be discontinued or not prior to investigation for PMB.
- There is unlikely to be any problem in histological interpretation if the patient remains on HRT provided the pathologist is given details of the hormonal treatment.
- On the other hand, stopping the HRT induces an oestrogen withdrawal bleed with loss of tissue that should be assessed.

Investigations

- Full blood count. Microcytic hypochromic anaemia with a low haemoglobin is a pointer towards a malignancy.
- Clotting screen.
- Check ESR and CRP if indicated.
- CA125 if suspicion of ovarian cancer.
- Blood sugar to exclude diabetes. Liver function tests (LFTs), urea and electrolytes (U&E), thyroid function test (TFT) – *only if indicated.*

One-stop clinics

Direct referral to a postmenopausal bleeding clinic is available in most regions. Such clinics provide a fast and efficient way of investigating PMB with access to several investigations such as ultrasound, endometrial sampling and hysteroscopy.

Transvaginal ultrasound (TVUS)

- TVUS is an initial screening tool for identifying which women are at a high and low risk of endometrial cancer.
- It is not diagnostic but a thickened endometrium is suggestive of pathology.[5]
- When ordered, the GP should request that the report includes the endometrial thickness; the GP should also state the menopausal status of the patient (e.g. pre-, peri- or post-).
- The threshold in the UK is 5 mm:
  — a thickness of <5 mm has a negative predictive value of 98%[3]
  — a thickness of >5 mm gives a 7.3% likelihood of endometrial cancer.[6]
- As some pathology may be missed, it is recommended that hysteroscopy and biopsy should be performed if clinical suspicion is high, irrespective of the endometrial thickness.[7]

Endometrial biopsy

- This can be obtained using an endometrial sampling device as an outpatient procedure.
- All methods of sampling will miss some cancers.[8,9]
- In a small proportion of patients, outpatient endometrial sampling will be technically impossible.
- It has a procedure failure rate and tissue-yield failure rate each of approximately 10%.[8,10]
- An adequate sample is more likely to be obtained if performed simultaneously with a hysteroscopy.
- As the false negative of endometrial sampling or biopsy is significant, current advice is that it should be combined with hysteroscopy.

Diagnostic hysteroscopy

- This is generally now available as an outpatient procedure in 'one stop' postmenopausal bleeding clinics.
- This is a highly specific, accurate and safe tool for detecting intrauterine abnormalities.
- It allows visualisation of an abnormal endometrium, indicates whether material for histological assessment is obtainable and may demonstrate the best method to achieve it.
- When endometrial sampling gives no yield, a negative hysteroscopy confirms that this outcome is acceptable.
- Hysteroscopy with biopsy is preferable. It is the first line of investigation in women taking tamoxifen as these women have a higher probability of malignancy (substantially >10%).[1]

Dilation and curettage (D&C)

Historically, endometrial samples have been obtained by D&C. However, as this technique is carried out blindly, endometrial lesions may be missed. One study showed that in 60% of patients less than half the cavity was curetted.[11]

D&C should no longer be used as the first-line method of investigating PMB. If undertaken, a concurrent hysteroscopy should be performed.

Treatment regime

Where pathology is found, treatment and prognosis will depend upon the condition. If no pathology is found, the patient is reassured and any symptomatic benign disease treated accordingly.

- If the pelvic examination is normal, bleeding has stopped and the endometrial thickness is <5 mm, no further action is needed.
- If the endometrial thickness is >5 mm, bleeding recurs or scan has identified polyp or submucous fibroid, referral for hysteroscopy is indicated.
- Hysteroscopy and curettage is the gold standard investigation as it allows visualisation of the uterine cavity and biopsy of the specific lesion.
- Vaginal atrophy can be treated with topical oestrogens. If other menopausal symptoms are present, HRT may be used (exclude contraindications).
- Endometrial polyps can be removed during hysteroscopy.
- Cervical polyps can be removed as an outpatient procedure. Any polyp removed must be sent for histology.
- Endometrial hyperplasia without atypia can be treated with progestogens. Complex endometrial hyperplasia with atypia should be treated as endometrial cancer.[12]
- Endometrial biopsy is performed to obtain a histological diagnosis. Endometrial cancer is staged based on surgical pathological findings – FIGO staging system (Table 11.1).

TABLE 11.1 FIGO staging system

Stage Ia and Ib	Total abdominal hysterectomy with bilateral salpingo-oophorectomy (TAH&BSO)
Stage Ic and stage II	Pelvic radiotherapy + surgery + lymph node dissection
Stage III	Surgery + external beam radiotherapy + intracavity radiotherapy
Stage IV	Radiotherapy + progestogens. Chemotherapy is also sometimes used[13]

GP surveillance

If endometrial thickness is <5 mm with no risk factors, the GP can observe; referral for endometrial biopsy must be done if further bleeding occurs.

Recurrent postmenopausal bleeding

There is no evidence to recommend when re-investigation should take place and therefore clinical judgement is required. As a precaution, re-investigation of recurrent PMB should be considered after 6 months.[1]

KEY POINTS

- Postmenopausal bleeding should signal malignancy until proven benign. All patients should be referred under the 2-week referral rule.
- Taking a good history is important as some women may not be able to differentiate between vaginal, urethral or a rectal blood loss.
- Women on tamoxifen should always have an endometrial biopsy as TVUS has been shown to be neither sensitive nor specific for neoplasia in these women.[5]
- If the patient is taking HRT, then an immediate referral may not be appropriate as bleeding or spotting is an expected side effect.
- A normal examination and endometrial thickness of <5 mm means no more action is required.
- Investigation is required if bleeding persists after the first 6 months of taking HRT or occurs after amenorrhoea has been established or if bleeding occurs outside the time of progestogen withdrawal in women on cyclical HRT.[14]
- A dedicated postmenopausal bleeding clinic in the familiar surroundings of primary care is the most appropriate cost-effective initial screen.

Useful websites

For patients – helplines

www.patient.co.uk

For GPs

RCOG women's health guidelines: www.rcog.org.uk/womens-health

Referral guidelines for suspected cancer—National Institute for Health and Clinical Excellence.; www.nice.org.uk/nicemedia/pdf/CG027quickrefguide.pdf

Uterine cancer: average number of new cases per year and age-specific incidence rates UK 2006–08: www.info.cancerresearchuk.org/cancerstats/types/uterus/incidence

Postmenopausal bleeding should be referred urgently. The Practitioner: www.theprac-titioner.co.uk/ewcommon/tools/download.ashx?doc1d

References

1 Scottish Intercollegiate Guidelines Network. Investigation of post-menopausal bleeding: a national clinical guideline. Edinburgh: SIGN; 2002.

2 Moodley M, Roberts C. Clinical pathway for the evaluation of postmenopausal bleeding with an emphasis on endometrial cancer detection. *J Obstet Gynaecol.* 2004 Oct; **24**(7): 736–41.

3 Sahdev A. Imaging the endometrium in postmenopausal bleeding. *BMJ.* 2007 Mar 24; **334**(7594): 635–6.

4 National Institute for Health and Clinical Excellence. Referral for Suspected Cancer: NICE guideline 27. London: NIHCE; 2005. www.nice.org.uk/CG27

5 Cancer Australia. Abnormal vaginal bleeding in pre-, peri- and postmeno-pausal women: a diagnostic guide for general practitioners and gynaecologists. Sydney: Cancer Australia; 2011. Available at: www.canceraustralia.gov.au/publications-resources/cancer-australia-publications/abnormal-vaginal-bleeding-pre-peri-and-post

6 Smith-Bindman R, Weiss E, Feldstein V. How thick is too thick? When endome-trial thickness should prompt biopsy in postmenopausal women without vaginal bleeding. *Ultrasound Obstet Gynecol.* 2004 Oct; **24**(5): 558–65.

7 Litta P, Merlin F, Saccardi C, *et al.* Role of hysteroscopy with endometrial biopsy to rule out endometrial cancer in postmenopausal women with abnormal uterine bleeding. *Maturitas.* 2005 Feb 14; **50**(2): 117–23.

8 Gordon SJ, Westgate J. The incidence and management of failed Pipelle sampling in a general outpatient clinic. *Aust NZ Obstet Gynaecol.* 1999; **39**(1): 115–18.

9 Tahir MM, Bigrigg MA, Browning JJ, *et al.* A randomised controlled trial com-paring transvaginal ultrasound, outpatient hysteroscopy and endometrial biopsy with inpatient hysteroscopy and curettage. *Br J Obstet Gynaecol.* 1999; **106**(12): 1259–64.

10 Etherington IJ, Harrison KR, Read MD. A comparison of outpatient endometrial sampling with hysteroscopy, curettage and cystoscopy in the evaluation of post-menopausal bleeding. *J Obstet Gynaecol.* 1995; 15: 259–62.

11 Stock RJ, Kanbour A. Prehysterectomy curettage. *Obstet Gynaecol.* 1975; **45**(5): 537–41.

12 Mongomery B, Daum G, Dunton C. Endometrial hyperplasia: a review. *Obstet Gynaecol Surv.* 2004; **59**(5): 368–78.

13 Hogberg T. Adjuvant chemotherapy in endometrial cancer. *Int J Gynecol Cancer.* 2010; **20**(11 Suppl 2): S57–9.

14 Spencer CP, Cooper AJ, Whitehead MI. Management of abnormal bleeding in women receiving hormone replacement therapy. *BMJ.* 1997; 315: 37–42.

Postcoital bleeding

DEFINITION

Postcoital bleeding (PCB) is non-menstrual bleeding that occurs immediately after sexual intercourse. It is more likely to originate from the vagina or cervix rather than the endometrium.

It is a symptom, not a diagnosis, and therefore warrants further investigation. The main aim of investigating PCB is to exclude cervical cancer.

Prevalence

PCB occurs in 0.7%–39% of women with cervical cancer.[1] The risk of cervical cancer in women presenting with PCB is approximately 1 in 44 000 in 20–24-year-olds and 1 in 2400 in 45–54-year-olds.[1]

In a study looking at pathological findings in a group of women attending colposcopy for PCB but with negative cervical smear, 33% had an ectropion, 12% had cervical polyps, 7% had cervical intraepithelial neoplasia (CIN) and 2% had chlamydia. However no pathology was found in 50% of the women and nobody in the study had invasive cancer.[2]

Aetiology

Cervical:
- infection – chlamydia, gonorrhea
- polyps – cervical, endometrial
- cervical ectropion
- trauma
- condylomata acuminata (genital warts)
- carcinoma.

Vaginal:
- trauma – during intercourse, sex toys, piercing
- vaginitis – infectious (*Candida*, bacterial vaginosis (BV), *Trichomonas vaginalis*, chlamydia, gonorrhoea)
- non-infectious – atrophic
- carcinoma – very rare.

Endometrial:
- polyps – if they hang through the cervix
- carcinoma.

Primary care management
History
Menstrual history:
- LMP – when and if normal
- normal cycle duration and length
- acute or chronic problem
- any menorrhagia?
- at what point in cycle does PCB occur?
- any bleeding following exercise?
- any associated symptoms (e.g. abdominal pain, fever, discharge)?
- establish bleeding is from the vagina, not rectum or in the urine.

Gynaecological history:
- current use of contraception
- smears: are they up to date?; most recent test results; any previous smear abnormalities and/or referral for colposcopy
- previous gynaecological surgery?

Sexual history:
- risk factors for STI – age <25 or any age with a new partner/more than one partner in the last year; previous STIs
- barrier contraception – is this always used?

Obstetric history:
- parity if applicable
- time since last delivery or pregnancy (miscarriage or termination)
- risk of current pregnancy, e.g. missed pills.

Examination
Abdominal: noting the presence/absence of pelvic masses.

Vaginal (speculum and bimanual): looking for obvious genital tract pathology, e.g. presence of ulceration, discharge or polyps. Eighty per cent of cervical cancer is diagnosed on speculum examination.[3]

- Cervical ectropion:
  - — common in pregnancy and in women taking the combined pill
  - — it appears as a red ring surrounding the external os as the less resilient columnar epithelium of the endocervix extends downwards, replacing the stratified squamous epithelium of the vaginal portion of the cervix.
- Cervical polyp:
  - — mass arising from the endocervix; occasionally endometrial polyps can be seen extruding through the os.
- Cervicitis:
  - — the cervix is tender, red and oedematous
  - — there may be mucopurulent discharge
  - — the most common cause currently is *Chlamydia trachomatis*. Other causes include *Neisseria gonorrhoeae*, *Trichomonas vaginalis*, herpes simplex and human papillomavirus (HPV).

Investigations[4]

Investigations should include:
- infection screening – always consider STIs, in particular chlamydia
- pregnancy test – if positive, urgent referral for USS +/– bHCG to exclude ectopic pregnancy
- cervical smear – should only be taken where a woman is due or overdue a smear.

Referral for further investigation

Colposcopy

Despite the low rate of serious pathologies in cases with a recent negative cervical smear, there remains some concern that these women are at increased risk of CIN and therefore warrant a colposcopy referral.[5]

Management

This will be dependent on the cause:
- Cervicitis:
  - — antibiotic treatment as appropriate, including contact tracing; refer to GUM if necessary
  - — electrocautery of secondary infected Nabothian follicles for chronic cervicitis.
- Cervical ectropion:
  - — these may resolve spontaneously after pregnancy or if the combined

pill is stopped (progesterone-only contraception may be used instead)

— refer gynaecology/colposcopy for treatment with silver nitrate cautery, cryocautery or diathermy.

- Cervical polyps:
  — polyps should always be removed and sent for histology. They can be avulsed at the surgery if on a stalk and haemostasis achieved with silver nitrate – however, broad-base polyps should be referred
  — they can be accompanied by endometrial polyps in 25%, so an ultrasound scan +/− hysteroscopy may be indicated, especially in older women.[6]
- Suspected cancer.[3] Urgent referral if:
  — on speculum examination there is a lesion suspicious of cancer on the cervix or vagina
  — on the clinical examination there is a lesion suspicious of cancer on the vulva
  — PCB persisting for more that 4 weeks in a woman aged >35; do not wait for a smear result
  — suspicious pelvic mass on pelvic examination.

These women should be seen urgently, within two weeks of referral and examination should be performed by a gynaecologist experienced in the management of cervical disease (such as a cancer lead gynaecologist).[7]

'Early' referral but not 'urgent': repeated unexplained postcoital bleeding.

KEY POINTS

- Women with PCB should have a cervical speculum examination at presentation to identify local causes of bleeding.
- A woman presenting with PCB who has negative cytology has a greatly reduced risk of cervical cancer but the risk is not totally eliminated.
- Urgent referral is necessary if clinical features are suggestive of cervical cancer on examination, irrespective of a previous negative smear result.
- Any clinical suspicion is an indication for referral and not for a cervical smear.[3]

Useful websites

For patients – helplines

www.patient.co.uk

For GPs

RCOG women's health guidelines: www.rcog.org.uk/womens-health

References

1 Shapley M, Jordan J, Croft PR. A systemic review of postcoital bleeding and risk of cervical cancer. *Br J Gen Pract.* 2006 Jun; **56**(527): 453–60.

2 Sahu B, Latheef R, Aboel Magd S. Prevalence of pathology in women attending colposcopy for postcoital bleeding with negative cervical cytology. *Arch Gynecol Obstet.* 2007 Nov; **276**(5): 471–3.

3 Scottish Executive. Scottish referral guidelines for suspected cancer. NHS; 2007. Available at: www.sehd.scot.nhs.uk/mels/HDL2007_09.pdf (accessed 14 December 2012).

4 Clinical Effectiveness Unit. Management of unscheduled bleeding in women using hormonal contraception. London: Faculty of Sexual and Reproductive Healthcare (RCOG); 2009. Available at: www.fsrh.org/pdfs/unscheduledbleedingmay09.pdf (accessed 14 December 2012).

5 Abu J, Davies Q, Ireland D. Should women with postcoital bleeding be referred for colposcopy? *J Obstet Gynaecol.* 2006 Jan; **26**(1): 45–7.

6 Stamatellos I, Stamatopoulos P, Bontis J. The role of hysteroscopy in the current management of the cervical polyps. *Arch Gynecol Obstet.* 2007 Oct; **276**(4): 299–303.

7 NHS Cancer Screening Programme. Colposcopy and programme management: guidelines for the NHS Cervical Screening Programme. 2nd ed. London: NHS; 2010.

13

Intermenstrual bleeding

> **DEFINITION**
>
> Intermenstrual bleeding (IMB) refers to vaginal bleeding at any time during the menstrual cycle other than during normal menstruation. It is a symptom, not a diagnosis, and therefore warrants further investigation.

Prevalence

Intermenstrual bleeding has an annual cumulative incidence of 17% in menstruating women as shown by a study based in a general practice setting.[1] Less than 5% of endometrial cancers occur in premenopausal women.[2]

Women with risk factors for endometrial cancer who present with IMB should be fully investigated. Risk factors for endometrial cancer include: nulliparity, exposure to unopposed oestrogen, obesity, polycystic ovary syndrome, the use of tamoxifen and strong family history of endometrial or colon cancer (Lynch syndrome).

Aetiology[3]

Contributing factors may include:

- Pregnancy-related factors including ectopic pregnancy.
- Physiological – 1%–2% spot around ovulation.
- Iatrogenic:
  — combined oral contraceptive pill (COCP), e.g. too low a dose, concurrent antiepileptic treatment or diarrhoea
  — progesterone-only pill
  — contraceptive depot injections (Depo-Provera)
  — intrauterine systems (IUS)[4] or implant

— emergency contraception[5]
— following smear or treatment to the cervix
— caesarean section scars[6]
— drugs altering clotting parameters, e.g. anticoagulants, selective serotonin reuptake inhibitors (SSRIs), corticosteroids
— tamoxifen
— alternative remedies, e.g. ginseng, ginkgo, soy supplements and St John's wort.[7]
- Vaginal causes:
  — adenosis
  — vaginitis (bleeding uncommon before the menopause)
  — tumours.
- Cervical causes:
  — infection – chlamydia, gonorrhoea
  — cancer (but bleeding is most often postcoital)
  — cervical polyps
  — cervical ectropion – can bleed spontaneously or after intercourse
  — condylomata acuminata of the cervix.
- Uterine causes:
  — endometrial polyps
  — endometritis, endometriosis
  — adenomyosis (usually symptomatic later in life)
  — cancer (endometrial adenocarcinoma, adenosarcoma[8] and leiomyosarcoma)
  — fibroids.
- Ovarian causes:
  — oestrogen-secreting ovarian cancers.

Primary care management

History

Menstrual history:
- last menstrual period (LMP) – when and if 'normal'
- what is the usual cycle duration and length?
- duration – long-standing problem or recent change?
- associated menorrhagia
- at what point in cycle does IMB occur?
- any bleeding following exercise?
- any associated symptoms? e.g abdominal pain, fever, discharge, dyspareunia
- aggravating factors, e.g. exercise, intercourse
- quality of life in relation to the IMB.

Obstetric history:

- parity
- time since last delivery or pregnancy (miscarriage or termination)
- current breastfeeding
- risk of current pregnancy, e.g. missed pills, unprotected intercourse
- risk factors for ectopic pregnancy – history of pelvic inflammatory disease or endometriosis, IVF treatment, IUCD in-situ.

Gynaecological history:

- current use of contraception
- smears: most recent test results; any previous smear abnormalities and/ or referral for colposcopy
- previous gynaecological investigations or surgery?

Medical history:

- diabetes
- bleeding disorders
- current medication, e.g. tamoxifen; over-the-counter herbal medicines.

Sexual history:

- risk factors for sexually transmitted infection (STI): age <25 or any age with a new partner/more than one partner in the last year; previous STIs
- barrier contraception – is this always used?

Examination

Abdominal:

- BMI: a high BMI is an independent risk factor for endometrial cancer.
- Note the presence/absence of pelvic masses.

Vaginal (speculum and bimanual):

- A full pelvic examination is mandatory, including a cervical speculum examination[9] and inspection of the vulva.
- Look for obvious genital tract pathology, e.g. contact bleeding, presence of ulceration, discharge or polyps.
- Cervical ectropion:
  — common in pregnancy and in women taking the combined pill
  — it appears as a red ring surrounding the external os.
- Cervical polyp:
  — mass arising from the endocervix; occasionally endometrial polyps can be seen extruding through the external os.

- Cervicitis:
  - cervix is tender, red, and oedematous
  - there may be mucopurulent discharge.

Investigations
- Infection screen: always consider STIs, in particular chlamydia.
- Pregnancy test – if positive, urgent referral for USS +/– bHCG to exclude ectopic pregnancy.
- Blood tests:
  - full blood count (FBC)
  - clotting screen
  - thyroid function if thyroid disorder suspected
  - FSH/LH levels (if onset of menopause suspected).

Referral for further investigation[10,11]
Refer for investigation if persistent IMB lasting 3 months or more and negative clinical findings in:
- women >45 years
- women aged <45 years with risk factors for endometrial cancer who have persistent IMB since >3 months of starting a contraceptive method
- women aged <45 years with risk factors for endometrial cancer who present with a change in bleeding pattern.

Transvaginal ultrasound (TVUS):
- Investigation of choice to look for structural abnormality.
- An endometrial thickness of 8 mm or less is significantly less likely to be associated with a malignant pathology.[12]
- Evidence of endometrial thickening should prompt referral for biopsy as pathology can be missed on ultrasound, particularly in the presence of an IUCD.[13]
- Interpretation of endometrial thickness in the premenopausal woman is dependent on the time of menstrual cycle during which the ultrasound is performed. The most accurate results are achieved if performed at the end of the period.[14]

Endometrial biopsy:
- May be performed as a surgery or clinic-based procedure, but these miss up to 18% of focal lesions.[3]
- Hysteroscopy with biopsy is the current gold standard for investigating the uterine cavity, allowing direct visualisation and tissue diagnosis.[15]

Diagnostic hysteroscopy:
- Should be performed if a TVUS is inconclusive or suggestive of intrauterine pathology.

Management
Management will be dependent on the cause, as outlined below.

Suspected cancer[2]
Urgent referral (within 2 weeks) if:
- on speculum examination there is a lesion suspicious of cancer on the cervix or vagina
- on the clinical examination there is a lesion suspicious of cancer on the vulva
- PCB persisting for more that 4 weeks in a woman aged >35; do not wait for a smear result
- suspicious pelvic mass on pelvic examination
- persistent IMB but negative examination findings.

Infection
- Antibiotic treatment as appropriate, including contact tracing. Refer to genitourinary medicine (GUM) if necessary.

Unscheduled bleeding with hormonal contraceptives[10]
- Before starting hormonal contraception, women should be advised that unscheduled bleeding is common in the first 3 months after starting a new hormonal contraceptive method and for up to 6 months with the IUS and progestogen-only implant. However, follow-up should be planned as bleeding may persist beyond this time.
- For persistent bleeding or change in bleeding pattern after 3 months of use, or where a woman has not participated in a National Cervical Screening Programme, a speculum +/– bimanual examination should be performed.

If using the combined oral contraceptive pill (COC):
- Continue with the same pill for at least 3 months, as bleeding often settles within this time.
- Use a pill with a dose of ethinylestradiol sufficient to provide the best cycle control – consider increasing to a maximum of 35 micrograms.
- Try a different pill or a different progestogen dose or type; may help on an individual basis.

If using the progesterone-only pill (POP):

- Trying a different POP may help on an individual basis (although little evidence that changing the progestogen dose or type improves bleeding).
- No evidence that desogestrel-only pills (e.g. Cerazette) have better bleeding patterns than traditional POPs.
- No evidence that using two POPs per day improves bleeding.

If using the progestogen-only implant, Depo-Provera or IUS:

- A first-line COCP (with 30–35 micrograms ethinylestradiol) may be considered for up to 3 months in the usual cyclical regimen or continuously without a pill-free interval (this is an unlicensed indication).
- No evidence that reducing the injection interval for Depo-Provera injections improves bleeding, but the injection can be given up to 2 weeks early.
- Mefenamic acid 500 mg twice or three times daily for 5 days can be used to reduce the duration of bleeding for women on Depo-Provera injections.

Reassure: if the patient is <45 years with normal clinical findings **and** no risk factors for endometrial cancer **and** no other associated symptoms, reassurance is the treatment.

KEY POINTS

- Always exclude pregnancy and STIs as a possible cause of bleeding.
- A full pelvic examination including speculum examination is mandatory for symptoms of intermenstrual and postcoital bleeding.
- Consider urgent referral for women with persistent IMB but negative examination findings.
- Any clinical suspicion is an indication for referral and not for a cervical smear.[2]

Useful websites

For patients – helplines

www.patient.co.uk

For GPs

RCOG women's health guidelines: www.rcog.org.uk/womens-health

References

1 Shapley M, Jordan K, Croft PR. An epidemiological survey of symptoms of menstrual loss in the community. *Br J Gen Pract*. 2004 May; **54**(502): 359–63.

2 Scottish Executive. Scottish referral guidelines for suspected cancer. NHS; 2007. Available at: www.sehd.scot.nhs.uk/mels/HDL2007_09.pdf (accessed 14 December 2012).

3 Albers JR, Hull SK, Wesley RM. Abnormal uterine bleeding. *Am Fam Physician*. 2004 Apr 15; **69**(8): 1915–26. [abstract]

4 Guttinger A, Critchley HO. Endometrial effects of intrauterine levonorgestrel. *Contraception*. 2007 Jun; **75**(6 Suppl): S93–8. Epub 2007 Mar 23. [abstract]

5 Gainer E, Kenfack B, Mboudou E, *et al*. Menstrual bleeding patterns following levonorgestrel emergency contraception. *Contraception*. 2006 Aug; **74**(2): 118–24. Epub 2006 Apr 27. [abstract]

6 Tahara M, Shimizu T, Shimoura H. Preliminary report of treatment with oral contraceptive pills for intermenstrual vaginal bleeding secondary to a cesarean section scar. *Fertil Steril*. 2006 Aug; **86**(2): 477–9. Epub 2006 Jun 12. [abstract]

7 Murphy PA, Kern SE, Stanczyk FZ, *et al*. Interaction of St. John's wort with oral contraceptives: effects on the pharmacokinetics of norethindrone and ethinyl estradiol, ovarian activity and breakthrough bleeding. *Contraception*. 2005 Jun; **71**(6): 402–8. [abstract]

8 Abu J, Ireland D, Brown L. Adenosarcoma of an endometrial polyp in a 27-year-old nulligravida: a case report. *J Reprod Med*. 2007 Apr; 52(4): 326–8. [abstract]

9 National Institute for Health and Clinical Excellence. Referral for Suspected Cancer: NICE guideline 27. London: NIHCE; 2005. www.nice.org.uk/CG27

10 Clinical Effectiveness Unit. Management of unscheduled bleeding in women using hormonal contraception. London: Faculty of Sexual and Reproductive Healthcare (RCOG); 2009. Available at: www.fsrh.org/pdfs/unscheduledbleedingmay09.pdf (accessed 14 December 2012).

11 National Institute for Health and Clinical Excellence. Heavy Menstrual Bleeding: NICE guideline 44. London: NIHCE; 2007. www.nice.org.uk/guidance/CG44

12 Getpook C, Wattanakumtornkul S. Endometrial thickness screening in premenopausal women with abnormal uterine bleeding. *J Obstet Gynaecol Res*. 2006 Dec; **32**(6): 588–92. [abstract]

13 Pitkin J. Dysfunctional uterine bleeding. *BMJ*. 2007 May 26; **334**(7603): 1110–11.

14 Cancer Australia. Abnormal vaginal bleeding in pre-, peri- and postmenopausal women: a diagnostic guide for general practitioners and gynaecologists. Sydney: Cancer Australia; 2011. Available at: www.canceraustralia.gov.au/publications-resources/cancer-australia-publications/abnormal-vaginal-bleeding-pre-peri-and-post

15 Naim NM, Mahdy ZA, Ahmad S, *et al*. The Vabra aspirator versus the Pipelle device for outpatient endometrial sampling. *Aust NZ J Obstet Gynaecol*. 2007 Apr; **47**(2): 132–6. [abstract]

14

Genital prolapse

> **DEFINITION**
>
> Genital prolapse or pelvic organ prolapse is defined as the descent of the pelvic organs into the vagina. It occurs when the pelvic muscles and connective tissues weaken.

Prevalence

The exact prevalence is unknown, as many women with prolapse do not consult a doctor. It is often asymptomatic and diagnosed during clinical examination as an incidental finding.[1] In the UK, prolapse accounts for 20% of women who are on the waiting list for major gynaecological surgery.[2]

Forty per cent of participants in the Women's Health Initiative (WHI) trial in the US had some degree of prolapse. Of the 27 342 women enrolled in the study, uterine prolapse was seen in 14%.[3]

The Oxford Family Planning Association study followed women in the age group 25–39 years and found the hospital admission with prolapse was 20.4 per 10 000 annually and the incidence of surgery for prolapse was 16.2 per 10 000 annually.[4]

Risk factors[5,6]

Risk factors for genital prolapse include:

- Menopause due to oestrogen deficiency: although menopause is a well-documented risk factor, a study of 270 women from the Women's Health Initiative (WHI) trial in the United States who had undergone hysterectomy found no association between oestrogen status and prolapse.[7]

- Age: the risk of prolapse increases with age.[8]
- Obesity: this creates extra pressure in the pelvic area.
- Pregnancy.
- Higher parity: it is rare in women who have not had children.
- Race: Caucasians are at greater risk. Africans, Americans and Asians are affected less often.
- Conditions which raise the intra-abdominal pressure like heavy lifting, manual work, constipation and chronic obstructive pulmonary disease (COPD).
- Congenitally short vagina.
- Vaginal delivery, forceps/ventouse delivery, long second stage of labour and episiotomy, multiple or large babies.
- Previous pelvic surgery such as hysterectomy, colposuspension or bladder repair.
- Pelvic tumours (rare).

Stages of prolapse[9]

Stage 0: No prolapse
Stage 1: The most distal portion of the prolapse is >1 cm above the level of the hymen (within the vagina)
Stage 2: The most distal portion of the prolapse is ≤1 cm proximal or distal to the hymen (descent to the introitus)
Stage 3: The most distal portion of the prolapse is >1 cm below the hymen but protrudes no further than 2 cm less than the total length of the vagina
Stage 4: The full length of the prolapse bulges out of the vagina

Classification

Anterior compartment:
Urethrocele   prolapse of urethra
Cystocele   prolapse of bladder
Cystourethrocele   prolapse of bladder and urethra

Middle compartment:
Uterine or vault descent
Enterocele (herniation of pouch of Douglas)

Posterior compartment:
Rectocele   prolapse of rectum

The most common type of prolapse is cystocele, followed by uterine and then rectocele.

Primary care management

History

Onset of prolapse, associated symptoms and trying to find a precipitating factor is the first step towards establishing a diagnosis.

1. Vaginal symptoms:
   - feeling of fullness/pressure in the vagina
   - feeling of discomfort/dragging feeling
   - bulge/protrusion/something coming down
   - vaginal discharge
   - bleeding caused by ulceration.
2. Bowel symptoms:
   - constipation
   - feeling of incomplete emptying
   - straining
   - faecal incontinence
   - history of use of laxatives.
3. Urinary symptoms:
   - frequency
   - urgency
   - stress incontinence
   - manual reduction of prolapse needed to pass urine
   - incomplete emptying.
4. Sexual symptoms:
   - dyspareunia
   - inability to have intercourse
   - urinary incontinence during sex.
5. Less common symptoms:
   - lower back pains
   - pelvic or abdominal pain
   - difficulty walking
   - emotional and psychological symptoms (impact on body image).

Remember the mnemonic of urethral diverticulum (three Ds):
   Dribbling, Dyspareunia and Dysuria

Examination

General

- height
- weight
- body mass index (BMI)
- blood pressure (*a good medical practice in case patient needs to go for pelvic surgery*).

Per abdominal

- feel for distended bladder
- abdominal mass.

Per vaginal

A vaginal prolapse can change in size during the day (often reduced in the morning and more palpable after standing for long periods throughout the day). Examination findings will also depend on the position in which the woman is examined. Prolapse is usually larger on standing due to the effect of gravity on the pelvic floor. Very few women are examined in a standing position; the patient should be examined in the left lateral position. A Sims speculum should be inserted to hold back the posterior vaginal wall. The patient should be asked to cough or strain to increase pressure in the abdomen. This should demonstrate descent of the anterior vaginal wall, indicative of a cystocele or urethral displacement. Holding back the anterior vaginal wall will demonstrate a rectocele.

Stage 3 or 4 prolapse can be diagnosed without internal examination as it will be visible outside the vaginal opening.

A rectal examination should be performed to confirm posterior wall prolapse and distinguish rectocele from enterocele.

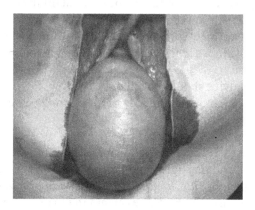

FIGURE 14.1 Vaginal prolapse

Exclude urethral diverticulum

The incidence of urethral diverticulum is between 0.6% and 5%. Most cases are probably secondary to obstetric urethral trauma or severe urethral infections.[10] It is an outpouching of urethral tissue into the space between the urethra and vagina.

Diagnosis is made on feeling a rounded cystic mass in the anterior wall of the vagina that leaks pus from the urethral orifice when pressure is applied.

Investigations

- Midstream urine (MSU) for culture and sensitivity analysis if patient has urinary symptoms.
- Intravenous pyelogram (IVP) if ureteral obstruction suspected due to complete prolapse.
- Cystometry and uroflowmetry if symptoms of urinary incontinence.
- Urodynamic studies.
- Ultrasound scan to exclude other pelvic problems.
- Magnetic resonance imaging (MRI) may be needed to image the pelvis if signs and symptoms do not correlate.
- MRI is the imaging modality of choice, if suspected urethral diverticulum.[11]

Treatment

Conservative

Conservative management must be offered to all patients by a primary care physician before referring the patient. Watchful waiting is most appropriate if prolapse is stage 1. These women must be examined at 4–6 monthly intervals to look for signs or development of new symptoms.

No consensus or evidence exists about whether we should intervene in the absence of symptoms, what should be the optimal timing of intervention, or whether early intervention reduces the incidence of recurrence.

The following treatment is recommended for women who have not completed their family, those who are not keen/suitable for surgery and those with mild prolapse.

The following advice should be offered.

- Weight management: advise if BMI >30. *Referral to a health trainer if available in your area.*
- Avoiding lifting heavy weights.
- High-fibre diet to avoid constipation and straining.
- Early diagnosis and management of asthma/COPD if persisting symptoms of cough. *This should not be difficult in primary care.*
- Pelvic floor exercises (PFE): these can aid the management of mild-degree prolapse and must always be encouraged postpartum during

postnatal examination. PFE can prevent the progression of prolapse and alleviate mild symptoms of prolapse.[12] They are not useful in stage 3 or stage 4 prolapse.[13] A Cochrane review of conservative management was published in 2006, concluding that there was no evidence from randomised controlled trials (RCTs) and that further trials were needed.[14] In recent studies some positive results have been shown with Colpexin Sphere.[15]

- Hormone replacement therapy (HRT): if the prolapse is related to menopause, HRT might be beneficial. Oestrogens in the HRT may help to strengthen the vaginal muscles.
- Antimuscarinic drugs like tolterodine can be an effective option in women with overactive bladder and concomitant mild anterior prolapse. A study from Italy assessed their effectiveness and found they are a good option.[16]
- Pessaries: vaginal pessaries have an established role in those who are not keen on surgery, are medically unfit for surgery and those waiting for surgery. The most commonly used are ring and shelf pessaries. In one study, the success rate with pessaries was 83%, with the highest rates occurring in those using HRT.[17] The aim should be to fit the largest pessary that does not cause discomfort. The common test is to sweep a finger between the pessary and walls of the vagina: if it can fit then the size of the pessary is right. Ask the patient to walk around, bend and micturate to ensure that the pessary is retained. There is no consensus as to how often a patient should be seen after a pessary is fitted successfully. At each follow up ask the patient about any symptoms and look for discharge or erosion. Complications related to pessary use are uncommon, the most common being vaginal infection, ulcerations, erosions or cystitis.[17]

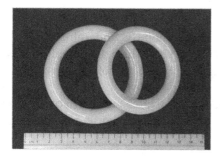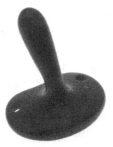

FIGURE 14.2 Ring pessary and shelf pessary

If you are thinking of providing a pessary service in primary care, please refer to Chapter 15, which describes how we achieved this in Oldham.

Urgent referral

Urgent referral if:

- complete procidentia
- vaginal ulceration
- urinary retention.

Surgical management

If conservative treatment is declined or ineffective, the patient should be referred to a urogynaecologist for surgical treatment.

Unfortunately the recurrence rate is higher after surgery. One study showed repeat surgery was needed in 29.2% of patients within 4 years of first surgery.[8] The life-time risk of prolapse surgery or incontinence by the age of 80 years has been reported as 11%.[6]

The main aims of surgical repair are:

- symptom control and better quality of life
- restoration of normal vaginal anatomy
- improvement of incontinence symptoms – bladder/bowel
- improvement of sexual function.

The choice of surgical option, whether abdominal or vaginal, depends upon the site, severity of prolapse and the general health of the woman.[8]

Uterine prolapse

- Vaginal hysterectomy is the treatment of choice.
- If cystocele or rectocele is present, hysterectomy is combined with anterior or posterior repair or both.
- Sacrohysteropexy is the treatment of choice in those who wish to retain the uterus.

Vaginal vault prolapse

- Laparoscopic and abdominal sacrocolpopexy. Abdominal sacrocolpopexy has a success rate of 90%. The main complications are intraoperative haemorrhage and a 3.3% risk of mesh erosion.[18] Laparoscopy results in a shorter hospital stay.
- Sacrospinous fixation and iliococcygeal hitch are alternative options. Abdominal incision is not required. Pain and shorter hospital stay are the main advantages.

Cystourethrocele

- Anterior repair with or without mesh via vaginal route is the treatment. Mesh may be placed in the anterior wall of the vagina for extra support.
  or

- Paravaginal repair is an abdominal approach to treat cystourethrocele. This procedure can also be done laparoscopically or vaginally.

Rectocele
- Posterior colporrhapy (posterior repair) with or without mesh.
- Perineoplasty and enterocele repair.
  or
- Sacrocolpopexy with mesh interposition via abdominal route.

Urethral diverticulum
Multiple techniques have been described for both open and endoscopic repair of the diverticulum.[19,20,21]

Postoperatively the patient should avoid heavy lifting, constipation and weight gain. She should be advised to avoid sexual intercourse for 6–8 weeks.

New surgical techniques
In recent years creating new surgical techniques has been at the forefront of pelvic organ prolapse management. Biological grafts include cadaveric fascia, human/porcine dermis and small intestine submucosa. Evidence from a recent Cochrane review suggested that the use of grafts or mesh inlays at the time of vaginal wall repair might reduce the risk of recurrent cystoceles.[22] The success rate of using synthetic meshes in anterior repairs has ranged from 42%[23] to 100%.[24] Biological grafts have also shown success in anterior and posterior repairs. Long-term data on success and complications are not available to support the use of mesh in vaginal surgery.

KEY POINTS

- The symptoms depend on the site and severity of prolapse.
- Initially patients should be assessed and managed conservatively by GPs.
- It is important to treat predisposing factors such as obesity, constipation and chronic obstructive pulmonary disease.
- Conservative treatment must be offered first: pelvic floor exercises for mild prolapse and vaginal pessary for patients unfit or unwilling for surgery.
- If conservative treatment is declined or is ineffective, the patient should be referred to secondary care.
- We do not know whether conservative management can prevent or delay the need for surgery and the best surgical approach to achieve anatomical cure, resolution of symptoms and low rate of recurrence.
- Recently there has been much interest in the use of mesh

augmentation to reduce the incidence of recurrence and to improve the outcome of the surgery.

Useful websites

For patients – helplines

Bladder and Bowel Foundation: www.bladderandbowelfoundation.org

Hysterectomy Association: www.hysterectomy-association.org.uk

Patient page on uterine prolapse: http://jama.ama-assn.org/cgi/reprint/293/16/2054.pdf

Prolapse. Wellbeing of Women. www.wellbeingofwomen.org.uk/your-wellbeing/your-health/prolapse/

Women's Health Concern: www.womens-health-concern.org

www.nhs.uk/Conditions/Prolapse-of-the-uterus/Pages/Causes.aspx

www.patient.co.uk/doctor/Genitourinary-prolapse.htm

For GPs

BMJ Clinical Evidence, genital prolapse in women: www.clinicalevidence.com/ceweb/condiions/who/0817/0817.jsp

Conservative management of pelvic organ prolapse in women: www.cochrane.org/reviews/en/ab003882/html

Mechanical devices for pelvic organ prolapse in women: www.cochrane.org/reviews/en/ab004010.html

Surgical management of pelvic organ prolapse in women: www.cochrane.org/reviews/en/ab/004014.html

References

1 Samuellson EC, Arne V, Tibblin G, *et al.* Signs of genital prolapse in a Swedish population of women 20 to 59 years of age and possible related factors. *Am J Obstet Gynecol.* 1999; **180**(2 Pt 1): 299–305.

2 Cardozo L. Prolapse. In: Whitefield CR, editor. *Dewhurst's Textbook of Obstetrics and Gynaecology for Postgraduates.* Oxford: Oxford Blackwell Science; 1995. pp. 642–52.

3 Hendrix SL, Clark A, Nygaard I, *et al.* Pelvic organ prolapse in the Women's Health Initiative: gravity and gravidity. *Am J Obstet Gynecol.* 2002; **186**(6): 1160–6.

4 Mant J, Painter R, Vessey M. Epidemiology of genital prolapse: observations from the Oxford Family Planning Association study. *Br J Obstet Gynaecol.* 1997; **104**(5): 579–85.

5 NHS Department of Health. 18 week commissioning pathway: pelvic organ prolapse. Version 4, June 2007. Available at: www.enfield.nhs.uk/local_services/gp_support/gp_18week_pathways/pathways_and_supplementary/pelvic_organ_prolapse.pdf (accessed 14 December 2012).

6 Olsen AL, Smith VJ, Bergstrom JO, *et al.* Epidemiology of surgically managed pelvic organ prolapse and urinary incontinence. *Obstet Gynecol.* 1997; **89**(4): 501–6.

7 Nygaard I, Bradley C, Brandt D. Pelvic organ prolapse in older women: prevalence and risk factors. *Obstet Gynecol.* 2004; **104**(3): 489–97.

8 Olsen AL, Smith VJ, Bergstrom JO, *et al.* Epidemiology of surgically managed pelvic organ prolapse and urinary incontinence. *Obstet Gynaecol.* 1997; **89**(4): 501–6.

9 Hall AF, Theofrastous JP, Cundiff GW, *et al.* Interobserver and intraobserver reliability of the proposed International Continence Society. Society of Gynecologic Surgeons and American Urogynecologic Society pelvic organ prolapse classification system. *Am J Obstet Gynecol.* 1996; **175**(6): 1467–70.

10 Tanagho EA, Brant WO, Lue TF. Disorders of the female urethra. In: Tanagho EA, McAninch JW, editors. *Smith's General Urology.* New York: McGraw-Hill; 2008. pp. 642–3.

11 Patel AK, Chapple CR. Female urethral diverticula. *Curr Opin Urol.* 2006; **16**(4): 248–54.

12 Davila GW, Bernier F. Multimodality pelvic physiotherapy treatment of urinary incontinence in adult women. *Int Urogynecol J.* 1995; 6: 187–94.

13 Dawila GW. Vaginal prolapse: management with nonsurgical techniques. *Postgrad Med.* 1996; **99**(4): 171–85.

14 Hagen S, Stark D, Maher C *et al.* Conservative management of pelvic organ prolapse in women. Cochrane Database Syst Rev. 2006; 4: CD003882.

15 Lukban JC, Aguirre OA, Davila GW, *et al.* Safety and effectiveness of Colpexin Sphere in the treatment of pelvic organ prolapse. *Int Urogynecol J Pelvic Floor Dysfunct.* 2006 Sep; **17**(5): 449–54.

16 Salvatore S, Serati M, Ghazzi F, *et al.* Efficacy of Tolterodine in women with detrusor overactivity and anterior vaginal wall prolapse: is it the same? *BJOG.* 2007 Nov **114**(11): 1436–8. Epub 2007.

17 Hanson LA, Schulz JA, Flood CG, *et al.* Vaginal pessaries in managing women with pelvic organ prolapse and urinary incontinence: patient characteristics and factors contributing to success. *Int Urogynecol J Pelvic Floor Dysfunct.* 2006 Feb; **17**(2): 155–9.

18 Fox SD, Stanton SL. Vault prolapse and rectocele: assessment of repair using sacrocolpopexy with mesh interposition. *BJOG.* 2000; **107**(11): 1371–5.

19 Lapides J. Transurethral treatment of urethral diverticula in women. *J Urol.* 1979; **121**(6): 736–8.

20 Moore TD. Diverticulum of the female urethra: an improved technique of surgical excision. *J Urol.* 1952; **68**(3): 611–6.

21 Wear JB. Urethral diverticulectomy in females. *Urol Times.* 1976; 4: 23.

22 Maher C, Baessier K, Glazener CM *et al.* Surgical management of pelvic organ prolapse in women. Cochrane Database Syst Rev. 2007; 3: CD004014.

23 Weber AM, Walters MD, Pledmonte MR. Anterior colporrhaphy: a randomised control trial of three surgical techniques. *Am J Obstet Gynecol.* 1996; 175: 10–17.

24 Flood CG, Drutz HP, Waja L. Anterior colporrhaphy reinforced with Marlex mesh for the treatment of cystoceles. *Int Urogynecol J Pelvic Floor Dysfunct.* 1998; **9**(4): 200–4.

15

Pessary service in NHS Oldham

Oldham Quality, Innovation, Productivity and Prevention Programme

One of the key measures of NHS Oldham's Quality, Innovation, Productivity and Prevention (QIPP) programme is the aim to minimise hospital follow-up appointments and treat patients more cost-effectively wherever possible. The resulting key performance indicators (KPIs) applied to provider contracts to reduce variation in follow-up activity levels led to the local Acute Trusts re-thinking their follow-up processes.

One consequence has been the local Acute Trust's decision to discharge (rather than arrange follow-ups) for patients requiring regular pessary changes – a service that can and should be delivered in a primary care setting. However, without primary care services in situ to meet demand, patients faced the prospect of seeking a GP referral each time they required their pessary changing, and the PCT faced a bill for hundreds of first appointments as opposed to follow-ups (more than double the cost).

As a Greater Manchester PCT, Oldham commissions gynaecology out-patient services from the Greater Manchester Clinical Assessment Service (GMCATS) – a Care UK service provided from mobile units at multiple locations across Greater Manchester.

However, as referral exclusion criteria apply to this service (BMI, co-morbidities, etc), it cannot treat everyone requiring this service. As a consultant-led service it would also not necessarily represent the best use of resources.

Another important factor was the 'guaranteed financial value' (GFV), or pre-paid level of the GMCATS contract – the PCT has a strong incentive to ensure this service is used up to a certain level of activity.

The proposed solution

Taking into account the following strategic priorities:

- patient choice;
- care closer to home;
- primary care capacity and capabilities.

The shadow Oldham Clinical Commissioning Group supported an intention to move towards an Any Qualified Provider (AQP) type model. This initially takes the form of a Local Enhanced Service (LES), which enables practices to become accredited to offer pessary services to patients registered with other Oldham practices. The medium term intention is to allow non-GP practice providers (e.g. sexual health service providers, district nursing services, etc.) to apply to become accredited pessary service providers through an open AQP tender process.

Inter-practice referral system

This service is the first in Oldham to involve a formalised intra-practice referral system that systematically builds in patient choice under a regulated framework. The model will soon also apply to minor surgery services. The shadow CCG is keen to realise the benefits and learning from these initiatives to inform strategy to release expertise residing in primary care through intra-practice referral systems in order to systematically ensure best value for money.

Better for patients

Women who need a change of pessary for vaginal prolapse will soon be able to choose from a number of practice-based services across Oldham and from GMCATS (if appropriate), if their registered GP practice does not already provide this service.

This pathway redesign will allow more women to be seen in the community, meaning they avoid unnecessary trips to hospital. It is expected that this will improve access and patient experiences and empower primary care clinicians who are able to carry out pessary fittings and changes.

Procedures will be carried out in a suitable clinical facility by trained and competent GPs and, in future, by other suitably qualified clinicians.

Policies and procedures

Practices that provide this service will be required to have a number of protocols and procedures in place, including infection control, consent policy, chaperone policy, patient leaflets, satisfaction and proper record keeping. They will also need to provide timely information to the patient's GP, along with any information relating to significant events that occur.

Provider activity levels and KPIs will be monitored through an Elective Care Performance Dashboard, generated via an in-house automated data collection and analysis system.

Patient leaflet about the ring pessary

The following template answers some of the common questions about the vaginal ring pessary. Patients are instructed to ask their doctor at the time of appointment if they would like more information.

What is a ring pessary?

This is a device shaped like a ring. It comes in various sizes and your size will be assessed by the doctor. This is inserted into the vagina by a trained doctor. The pessary is used to hold prolapse in place and relieve some of your symptoms related to prolapse.

Why do I need a ring pessary?

This has been suggested to you to relieve your symptoms of prolapse because/ you are unfit for surgery/you could be waiting for surgery/you have decided not to undergo the surgical procedure.

What happens during the appointment?

The doctor will ask you some questions related to prolapse. You will be asked to give your consent for the ring change either verbally or in writing. The old ring pessary will be removed by inserting a finger. A speculum will then be carefully inserted to examine the vaginal walls for any abnormality. After this a new pessary will be inserted using a lubricant gel/cream. You will be asked to move around, sit down and pass urine before you leave the clinic to make sure that the pessary is comfortable. Latex allergy is not a contraindication as most pessaries are silicone.

About the doctor

The doctor is a GP and is specially trained to do this procedure.

Risks/side effects

The procedure can cause some discomfort during removal and insertion but it is not painful. Vaginal infection is a common side effect which can be diagnosed and treated easily. Bladder infection, constipation, vaginal erosions, pain, bleeding, failure to reduce the prolapse and expulsion are some uncommon side effects.

Will the pessary affect my sexual life?
It is possible to have a normal sex life, although your partner may feel the pessary.

Will the pessary interfere with my going to the toilet?
No, it will not affect your bowels.

Will my pessary fall out?
After insertion the doctor will ask you to move about, cough and bear down to make sure that the pessary is of the right size. If the pessary falls out when you go home, please contact the surgery and a new pessary will be fitted.

How often does it need replacing?
Every 4 months. An appointment will be given at the time of insertion for change. You can always ring earlier than planned if any problems/side effects.

Follow-up appointment
The doctor will ask you some questions regarding any bleeding, vaginal discharge, bowel problems or urinary symptoms. With your consent an old pessary will be removed and a new one inserted. A new ring will not be inserted if there is vaginal ulcer or infection. You will be given a satisfaction questionnaire to fill.

Name of the doctor who has fitted the pessary:

Telephone no:

Please ring the surgery to cancel your appointment if you are unable to attend so that the appointment can be offered to someone else.

Summary of chaperone policy
The privacy and dignity needs of patients must be respected at all times and the needs of the patient, healthcare professional and the examination required will dictate the role of the chaperone.
1. Details of the examination, including the presence/absence/availability

of the chaperone and information given must be documented in the patient's case notes.

2. Ideally a chaperone should be a clinical health professional or trained non-clinical staff member who is:
   - sensitive and respectful of the patient's dignity and confidentiality
   - prepared to reassure the patient if they show signs of distress or discomfort
   - familiar with the procedures involved in the procedure or examination
   - prepared to raise concerns about the healthcare professional if misconduct occurs
   - ideally be the same sex as the patient
   - ideally be able to liaise with the patient in a common language.

16

Infertility

> **DEFINITION**
>
> **Primary infertility**: failure to conceive after two years of regular unprotected sexual intercourse in the absence of known reproductive pathology.
>
> **Secondary infertility**: as above, except that an initial pregnancy (including spontaneous or induced abortions) has occurred.

Prevalence

Eighty-four per cent of couples in the general population will conceive within 1 year if they have regular sexual intercourse. Those who fail in the first year will have a cumulative pregnancy rate of 92% by the second year.[1] With regular sexual intercourse, 94% of fertile women aged 35 years and 77% of women aged 38 years will conceive after 3 years.[1]

Causes[2]
Ovulatory causes
Anovulation (absent ovulation) or oligo-ovulation (infrequent ovulation) due to:
- polycystic ovarian syndrome (PCOS): commonest cause – 70% of all cases
- hypothalamic dysfunction
- hyperprolactinaemia
- age-related ovarian dysfunction
- premature ovarian failure.

TABLE 16.1 Causes of infertility

CAUSE	FREQUENCY
Ovulatory	25%
Tubal	20%
Uterine	<1%
Endometriosis	5%
Cervical	3%
Coital	5%
More than one cause	15%
Unexplained	25%
Male	30%

Tubal causes

Complete or partial blockage of fallopian tubes or due to peri-tubal adhesions caused by:

- sexually transmitted disease:
  - pelvic inflammatory disease (PID): infertility occurred in 8% of patients with one episode of PID, rising to 20% with two episodes and 40% in those with three or more episodes.[3] Infertility was higher following non-gonococcal PID (17%) than gonococcal PID (6%)[4]
  - endometriosis
- surgical intervention for management of ectopic pregnancy or other intra-abdominal condition
- non-gynaecological abdomino-pelvic infection
- congenital anomaly.

Uterine/peritoneal causes

Uterine/peritoneal causes include:
- intrauterine adhesions, polyps, fibroids
- abnormally shaped uterine cavity
- endometriosis.

Male factor infertility

Azoospermia (total absence of sperm) and oligospermia (reduced sperm numbers) due to:
- genetic disorders (Klinefelter's syndrome)
- genitourinary infections
- environmental factors such as medication, drugs, alcohol, smoking, radiation
- varicocoele, retrograde ejaculation, other hormonal problems, etc.

Unexplained infertility

Most investigations are normal. Various causes could be:

- problems with egg quality
- undiagnosed tubal dysfunction
- implantation failure.

Primary care management

History

Both partners:

- age (most important determinant of couple's fertility is the woman's age)
- duration of infertility
- previous fertility with different partners
- coital frequency, difficulties and timing
- medical-endocrine disorders (diabetes, thyroid problems)
- previous history of PID
- social history: history of smoking, alcohol, drug abuse, increasing weight
- occupation.

A case referent study investigated the relation between male infertility and occupational exposure, particularly glycol ethers. The study concluded that glycol ether exposure was related to low sperm count in men attending fertility clinics.[5]

Female:

- menstrual history
- previous contraception
- previous pregnancy
- galactorrhoea
- abdominal, pelvic or cervical surgery.

Male: mumps, orchitis, groin or genital surgery.

Examination

Both partners: height, weight, BMI and blood pressure.

Female:

General examination:

- fat and hair distribution
- breasts – galactorrhoea.

Bimanual examination:
- size of uterus
- mobility, adnexal
- masses/tenderness.

Speculum examination:
- vaginal septa/infections
- cervix – ectopy, polyps.

Male: genitalia-testicular size, varicocoele, hydrocoele.

Investigations
Female
- Mid-luteal progesterone levels predict ovulation. They are measured 7 days before the period (day 21 if cycle length is 28 days, day 28 if the cycle length is 35 days). Value of >30 nmol/l is proof of adequate ovulation.
- FSH/LH, oestradiol levels measurement on days 2–5 of menstrual cycle with day 1 being the first day of menstrual flow.
- Prolactin.
- Thyroid function test (TFT).
- Full blood count, serum ferritin, B12 level.
- Liver function test if suspected of alcohol abuse.
- Fasting blood sugar if clinically indicated.
- Pelvic ultrasound scan: only if clinically indicated. This is not a part of routine work up.
- Full screening for sexually transmitted infections (STIs).

Male
Semen analysis is usually requested in primary care. Any abnormality should prompt a referral for a repeat test within 3 months. A repeat test should be requested as soon as possible if there is azoospermia.

Semen analysis
Semen analysis is important but unfortunately it does not give a clear indication of whether the man has a fertility problem. A normal semen does not necessarily mean the man is fertile. An abnormal semen result is an indication of referral to a specialist.[6] The referral should be either to a clinical andrologist or a urologist. The specialist will be able to decide whether the problem is treatable or whether the patient needs assisted conception advice.[7] In a suboptimal sperm test, a further sample should be examined 12 weeks after the first sample as per World Health Organization (WHO)

guidelines on male fertility investigations. This will give a clear indication as to whether the semen is normal or not.[6]

TABLE 16.2 WHO normal reference values[8]

SEMEN ANALYSIS	
WHO normal reference values	
Volume	2.0 mL or more
pH	7.2–8.0
Sperm concentration	20 × 106 spermatozoa/mL or more
Total sperm count	40 × 106 spermatozoa per ejaculate
Motility	50% or more with forward progression (type a and b) or 25% or more with rapid progression (category a) within 60 minutes of ejaculation
Morphology	30% or more
Vitality	75% or more
White blood cells	Less than 1 × 106/mL
Immunobead test	Less than 20% spermatozoa with adherent particles
MAR test	Less than 10% spermatozoa with adherent particles

Further investigations

Likely to be carried out in secondary care

Tests for tubal patency:

1. Hysterosalpingogram (HSG): this is the investigation of choice unless there is history of pelvic inflammatory disease, previous ectopic pregnancy or endometriosis. A dye is passed into the womb and its passage through the tubes is monitored by X-ray. It is cheaper than laparoscopy and dye test. HSG is considered a safe and non-invasive procedure but it can be painful. Researchers randomised 200 infertile women undergoing this procedure to use either room temperature medium or medium pre-warmed to 37 degrees. Vasovagal episodes and a visual analogue of pain scale during HCG showed that warm contrast medium alleviated pain and significantly reduced the vasovagal episodes (8 versus 26, P = 0.001).[23]

2. Hysterosalpingo-contrast ultrasonography: this is the same as HSG but instead of X-ray, an ultrasound is used to monitor the passage of dye.

3. Laparoscopy and dye test: this test is usually indicated if there is a history of co-morbidities such as pelvic inflammatory disease or endometriosis. This emphasises the value of good history taking in primary care. It can also help evaluate the pelvis.

4. Hysterosalpingo contrast sonography, falloscopy and salpingoscopy – only performed in specialised fertility centres.

Treatment
Treatment focuses on the cause.

General advice

- Lifestyle advice: couples should be encouraged to pursue a healthy lifestyle – reducing alcohol intake, (less than 1–2 units per week in women and less than 3–4 units per week in men), stopping smoking, avoiding recreational drugs and maintaining a good diet. Men should be advised to avoid wearing tight underwear, having hot baths and avoiding any toxic chemicals (may not always be possible).
- Weight loss can significantly improve the chances of conception, especially in patients with polycystic ovarian disease (PCOS). The exact reason for this is uncertain although it may be linked to problems with insulin metabolism. Ideal BMI is 19–29 kg/m². In overweight or obese anovulatory women who wish to conceive, the first line of treatment is implementation of diet and lifestyle changes.[9] There is ample evidence that as little as 5%–10% reduction in body weight greatly improves the induction of ovulation.[10] Obesity BMI is >30 kg/m², or >25 kg/m² in women from south Asia; waist circumference >80 cm.[11]
- Discuss timing of intercourse and advise using a basal body temperature chart or an ovulation prediction kit.
- Preconceptional folic acid 400 µg and continue intake until first trimester.
- Rubella vaccination if indicated and advice on contraception for a month post vaccination.
- Cervical screening in accordance with the national screening programme.
- Psychological support and counselling to the couple.[2]
- Advise male partner to take antioxidant therapy to see if this improves quality of sperm. A new study found that men taking antioxidants were 4 times more likely to get their partners pregnant.[12] The most potent antioxidants are vitamin C 1000 mg with zinc and vitamin E.

Referral to secondary care

The Human Fertilisation and Embryology Authority recommends referral to centres that provide licensed treatments. GPs should be aware of these specialised clinics in their area.

Early referral

Female

Consider early referral if:
- aged over 35 years
- history of amenorrhoea/oligomenorrhoea:
  — polycystic ovarian syndrome (PCOS)
  — abnormal follicle stimulating/luteinising hormone
- previous abdominal/pelvic surgery
- previous pelvic inflammatory disease
- abnormal pelvic examination.

Male

Consider early referral if:
- previous genital pathology
- previous urogenital surgery
- previous sexually transmitted infection
- varicocoele
- significant systemic illness
- abnormal genital examination – undescended testis: oligospermia or azoospermia.

Treatment

Treatment depends on the cause of infertility.

Principle of treatment

The one and only one principle of fertility treatment is that the interests of the unborn child must be foremost.

Anovulatory infertility

Patients with normogonadotrophic anovulation (PCOS) are usually treated initially with clomiphene. If this does not work then the recommended treatment is metformin, gonadotrophins or ovarian drilling to increase ovulation. These treatments should not be initiated in primary care. Clomiphene can cause multiple pregnancies and so regular scanning is necessary during treatment. Metformin also should be used in a dedicated secondary care fertility clinic where its effectiveness can be accurately assessed. In cases of hypogonadotrophic hypogonadism, treatment with pulsatile GnRH agonists or gonadotrophin with luteinising activity has been found to be better in inducing ovulation. One trial compared the metabolic and reproductive effects of metformin, clomiphene and combination therapy. The authors concluded that clomiphene should be the first-line drug in women with PCOS. For those who have inadequate response, combination therapy can be tried before more invasive treatment is chosen.[13]

Patients with PCOS who have worse insulin sensitivity have a better ovulatory response to metformin, as compared to those with better insulin sensitivity who are more likely to respond to clomiphene.[14] Common side effects of clomiphene are: hot flushes, abdominal discomfort, multiple pregnancy, alopecia, ovarian enlargement, cyst formation.[15]

Tubal infertility

In vitro fertilisation (IVF) has replaced tubal surgery. It is estimated that live birth rates after tubal surgery range from 9%–69% depending on the severity of tubal disease – a poor outcome in those with severe tubal damage.[16] Selective salpingography plus tubal catheterisation or hysteroscopic tubal cannulation is the treatment of choice in women with proximal tubal obstruction.[1] One study found that the cumulative delivery rate after 72 months was 52% in the IVF group as compared to 59.5% in those who had tubal reversal.[17] The author concluded that surgical reversal is recommended for younger patients <37 years.

Uterine/peritoneal factor infertility

In minimal or mild endometriosis, ablation of endometriotic lesions and adhesiolysis is effective. Moderate and severe endometriosis should also be treated surgically, but often IVF will be necessary. NICE recommends surgical treatment of endometriosis for all severity of disease.[1]

Male factor infertility

Varicocoele treatment has proven not to be effective. In mild to moderate male infertility, intrauterine insemination (IUI) may be the first choice of treatment if semen preparation yields at least 1 million motile sperm and if morphology is above 5%. IVF and intracytoplasmic sperm injection (ICSI) are preferred for severe cases. Where there is low sperm quality, fertilisation rate may be low.[18] Certain centres may provide newer technologies such as the study of embryo cell division rates and greatly enhanced sperm morphological assessment. In severe male infertility, partial zonal dissection may result in a better outcome.[19]

Unexplained infertility: treatments
- Clomiphene treatment.
- Intrauterine insemination (IUI).
- In vitro fertilisation (IVF). A Cochrane review of IVF suggests that studies investigating this are limited by small sample size and that live birth rates have not been reported. For older women IVF may be the best option.[20]
- Perturbation treatment.[21]

Assisted conception treatments
Assisted conception can cause ovarian hyperstimulation syndrome. The procedure involves surgical intervention, so there is a risk of damage to pelvic organs or other structures within the pelvis.

Techniques developed in last three decades include:
- intrauterine insemination (IUI)
- in vitro fertilisation (IVF)
- intracytoplasmic sperm injection (ICSI)
- donor insemination
- oocyte donation.

Risks of fertility treatment
The regulatory body for assisted conception – the Human Fertilisation and Embryology Authority – is advocating the move to a single-embryo transfer to reduce the risk of multiple pregnancies:
- risk of failure
- risk of multiple pregnancies
- increased risk of foetal anomalies, cerebral palsy
- premature labour
- ovarian hyperstimulation due to assisted conception
- ovarian cancer caused by ovarian stimulation. There are conflicting studies.[22]

KEY POINTS

- Around 10% of couples are affected by infertility.
- The most important determinant of a couple's infertility is the woman's age.
- Lifestyle has a profound effect on fertility: obesity, smoking, alcohol and recreational drugs negatively affect the chance of conception.
- Infertility patients require a comprehensive investigation by knowledgeable physicians.

- The role of the GP is to initiate investigations for both partners and ensure timely referral to a dedicated specialist fertility clinic.
  - In a suboptimal sperm test, it is useful to do a repeat semen analysis 12 weeks after the first sample which is a full spermatogenesis cycle.
  - NICE recommends a stratified treatment approach for couples with unexplained infertility.
- The major treatment modalities for infertility are controlled ovarian stimulation with IUI for ovarian problems and unexplained infertility, surgery for selected patients with pelvic adhesions, endometriosis, etc. and IVF for patients with severe tubal disease, significant male factor infertility or failure to conceive with standard treatments.
  - With infertility treatment there is always a risk of failure, multiple pregnancies and foetal anomalies.
  - IVF, although it is the most invasive and immediately expensive procedure, is the most successful and is viewed as the most cost-effective option. This can only be achieved by appropriate funding.

Useful websites
For GPs
World Health Organization, Department of Reproductive Health and Research. *Laboratory Manual for the Examination and Processing of Human Semen.* 5th edition. Geneva: WHO; 2010. Available at: www.who.int/reproductivehealth/publications/infertility/9789241547789/en/index.html (accessed 15 December 2012).
Infertility Network UK: www.Infertilitynetworkuk.com

References
1 National Institute for Health and Clinical Excellence. Fertility: Assessment and Treatment for People with Fertility Problems: NICE guideline 11. London: NIHCE; 2004. http://publications.nice.org.uk/fertility-cg11

2 Hull MG, Glazener CM, Kelly NJ, *et al.* Population study of causes, treatment, and outcome of infertility. *BMJ. Clin Res Ed.* 1985; **291**(6510): 1693–7.

3 Westrom L. Effect of acute pelvic inflammatory disease on fertility. *Am J Obstet Gynecol.* 1975; 121: 707–13.

4 Westrom L, Joesoef MR, Reynolds GH, *et al.* Pelvic inflammatory disease and fertility. *Sex Transm Dis.* 1992; **19**(4): 185–92.

5 N Cherry, H Moore, R McNamee, *et al.* Occupation and male infertility: glycol ethers and other exposures. *Occup Environ Med.* 2008; **65**(10): 708–14.

6 World Health Organization. *Laboratory Manual for the Examination of Human Semen and Sperm: cervical mucus interaction.* 4th edition. Geneva: WHO; 1999.

7 Balen A. *Infertility in Practice.* 3rd edition. London: Informa Healthcare; 2008.

8 World Health Organization, Department of Reproductive Health and Research. *Laboratory Manual for the Examination and Processing of Human Semen*. 5th edition. Geneva: WHO; 2010. Available at: www.who.int/reproductivehealth/publications/infertility/9789241547789/en/index.html (accessed 15 December 2012).

9 Thessaloniki ESHRE/ASRM-sponsored PCOS consensus workshop group. Consensus on infertility treatment related to polycystic ovary syndrome. *Hum Reprod*. 2008; **23**(3): 462–77.

10 Clark AM, Ledger W, Galletly C, *et al*. Weight loss results in significant improvement in pregnancy and ovulation rates in anovulatory obese women. *Hum Reprod*. 1995; **10**(10); 2705–12.

11 National Institute for Health and Clinical Excellence. Obesity: The Prevention, Identification, Assessment and Management of Overweight and Obesity in Adults and Children: NICE guideline 43. London: NIHCE; 2006. www.nice.org.uk/CG43

12 Conley M. Antioxidants may increase male fertility. *ABC News*. 19 January 2011. Available at: http://abcnews.go.com/Health/antioxidants-increase-male-fertility/story?id=12641649#.UMuJhUZQt1M (accessed 15 December 2012).

13 Legro RS, Barnhart HX, Schlaff WD, *et al*. Clomiphene, metformin, or both for infertility in the polycystic ovary syndrome. *N Engl J Med*. 2007; 356: 551–66.

14 Palomba S, Falbo A, Orio F, *et al*. Efficacy predictors for metformin and clomiphene citrate treatment in anovulatory infertile patients with polycystic ovary syndrome. *Fertil Steril*. 2009; **91**(6): 2557–67.

15 British National Formulary (BNF). 63 March 2012. www.bnf.org

16 Pandian Z, Akanda VA, Harrid K *et al*. Surgery for tubal infertility. Cochrane Database Syst Rev. 2008; 3: CD064415.

17 Boeckxstaens A, Devroey P, Collins J, *et al*. Getting pregnant after tubal sterilisation: surgical reversal or IVF? *Hum Reprod*. 2007; **22**(10): 2660–4.

18 Trummer H, Caruso AP, Lipshultz LI, *et al*. Recent developments in the evaluation and treatment of male infertility. *Infect Urol*. 2000; 13: 87–94.

19 Schlegel PN, Girardi SK. Clinical review 87: in vitro fertilisation for male factor infertility. *J Clin Endocrinol Metab*. 1997; **82**(3): 709–16.

20 Tsafrir A, Simon A, Margalioth EJ, *et al*. What should be the first-line treatment for unexplained infertility in women over 40 years of age? *Reprod Biomed Online*. 2009; **19**(Suppl 4): 4334.

21 Edelstam G, Sjosten A, Bjuresten K, *et al*. A new rapid and effective method for treatment of unexplained infertility. *Hum Reprod*. 2008; **23**(4): 852–6.

22 Van Leeuwen FE, Klip H, Mooij T, *et al*. Risk of borderline and invasive ovarian tumours after ovarian stimulation for in vitro fertilisation in a large Dutch cohort. *Hum Reprod*. 2011; **26**(12): 3456–65.

23 Yi-Yang Zhu, Ying-Zi Mao, Wei-Ling Wu. Comparison of warm and cold contrast media for hysterosalpingography: a prospective randomized study. *Fertility and Sterility*. 2012; **97**(6): 1405–9.

REFERRAL GUIDE: Subfertility

Clinical presentation
- Failure to conceive after trying for 12 months in absence of known reproductive pathology
- Predisposing factors – amenorrhoea/oligomenorrhoea/pelvic inflammatory disease
- Woman's age >35 years

History
- Primary or secondary subfertility
- Menstrual cycle
- Sexual history
- Pregnancy history (secondary subfertility)
- Cervical screening history
- Associated medical problems
- Smoking/alcohol/use of recreational drugs

Examination
- BMI
- Blood pressure
- Abdominal examination
- Speculum and bimanual pelvic examination findings

Investigations
- HVS and endocervical swabs
- Rubella status
- Serum progesterone – a week before the expected period (day 21 for 28-day cycle; day 28 for 35-day cycle)
- Irregular and infrequent periods – FSH, LH and serum oestradiol
- Serum testosterone/androgen index in suspected cases of PCOS
- Serum prolactin for women – offered for women with suspected ovulatory disorder/women complaining of galactorrhoea
- Thyroid function tests
- Transvaginal scan

Primary/community provision prior to specialist opinion (unless indication for early referral)
- Women with BMI >25 (including women with diagnosed PCO) – given information about lifestyle management or referred to weight-monitoring clinic
- Help with smoking cessation and alcohol-related problems

- Positive chlamydial screening referred to appropriate clinic
- Women with amenorrhoea – investigated and offered progesterone challenge test
- Blood tests – if necessary repeated tests to check serum progesterone
- Psychosexual problems referred to community team for help

Indication for referral for specialist opinion

- Predisposing factors
- Pelvic or abdominal mass

17

Female urinary incontinence

Urinary incontinence is a common and distressing condition. It is an under-reported problem because of the stigma associated with the condition and many patients simply suffer in silence.

DEFINITION

Urinary incontinence is defined as involuntary leakage of urine.

Prevalence

It has been estimated that in the UK 9.6 million women are affected by bladder problems.[1,2] Overactive bladder itself affects 5 million adults, nearly 1 in 5 of the over-40 population.[3] Prevalence is estimated to be 15% among healthy older adults and 65% among older frail adults.[4] It is twice as high in women as in men. It can affect women of all ages including women post childbirth. In a cross-sectional survey of adult females attending a primary care practice in the UK, nearly half had urinary incontinence but only a small minority sought help.[5] Forty-two per cent of women affected wait up to 15 years before seeking treatment.[6]

Types

1. Stress incontinence

   This is an involuntary urine leakage on exertion such as coughing/laughing/sneezing or exercise. Stress incontinence is due to incompetent urethral sphincter. It is largely caused by childbirth, meaning young women can develop this problem. Other causes include pelvic surgery or hysterectomy.

2. Urge incontinence

This is an involuntary urinary leakage associated with urgency (a compelling desire to urinate that is difficult to defer) and is due to detrusor overactivity leading to detrusor contraction. Urge incontinence often appears later in life. Frequency or nocturia, with low volume of urine voided, are signs of overactive bladder which can occur with or without urge incontinence.[7] Overactive bladder affects both men and women and prevalence rises with age, affecting 16.7% of those aged 40 years in North America and Europe.[3] Overactive bladder should be managed in the same manner as urge incontinence.

3. Overflow incontinence

This is defined as the involuntary loss of urine associated with bladder over-distension in the absence of detrusor contraction. In women this is a relatively uncommon cause of urinary incontinence. Patients with overflow incontinence are at risk of urinary tract infection. The most common causes are advanced vaginal prolapse, postoperative obstruction if the bladder neck is overcorrected and spinal cord injury causing bladder hyporeflexia. Patients usually complain of loss of urine without awareness and constant wet feeling. Some women complain of sensation of full bladder and the need to strain to empty the bladder.

4. Mixed incontinence

This is both stress and urge incontinence.

Other useful definitions

- **Frequency**: a need to urinate many times during the day and/or night, normal or less than normal volumes of urine. This is due to the decrease in the capacity of bladder to hold urine. The normal range of passing urine varies from patient to patient. A normal range may be twice a night. Passing urine 6–7 times in one whole day is normal. Passing urine more than eight times in 24 hours is defined as frequent.
- **Nocturia**: the complaint that the individual has to wake up at night one or more times to empty bladder.
- **Polyuria**: polyuria involves urinating greater than 3 L per day.
- **Detrusor overactivity** (DO): this is a urodynamic diagnosis based on the observation of involuntary detrusor contractions during the filling phase of the bladder.
- **Urgency**: this is sudden compelling desire to pass urine which is difficult to defer.
- **Overactive bladder** (OAB) is a syndrome comprising symptoms of urgency with or without incontinence, usually with frequency and nocturia. The diagnosis and severity of the problem is determined by its impact on quality of life. The prevalence of OAB varies[8] depending

on population assessed and definitions used.[9] The prevalence increases with age owing to neurological and musculoskeletal effects, diabetes, congestive cardiac failure, cerebro-vascular accidents and medical therapy.

Risk factors

The incidence is higher in females. Other risk factors include:
- obesity
- elderly: urge incontinence increases with age
- pregnancy and childbirth
- obstruction; tumours in the pelvis, impacted stool
- hysterectomy[10]
- neurological disease
- cognitive impairment
- postmenopausal

Some useful facts
- Stress urinary incontinence is the commonest type of urinary incontinence.
- Normal functional bladder capacity for an adult female is between 350–700 ml.
- Palpable bladder tends to contain more than 200 ml residual urine.
- The residual volume should not be more than 150 ml.

Total incontinence related expenditure was more than £420 million in 2002 in UK, with the NHS purchasing £80 million worth of absorbent products alone (Royal College of Nursing). The cost estimated by the Bladder and Bowel Foundation (2010) in England is £7178.[11] It is expected to be much higher now. Only a small proportion of the above amount was spent on drugs[12] – the remainder was spent on secondary care and surgical treatment.

Bearing this in mind, GPs are ideally placed to screen and manage these patients within primary care. It is not necessary to refer *all patients* to secondary care. Now, with ever-increasing pressure on GPs to reduce unnecessary referrals, there is scope for commissioning this service. The management of overactive bladder is not a part of the Quality and Outcomes Framework, which could be a reason why GPs are not enthusiastic.

Primary care management

History

The history taking makes the initial diagnosis.

- Ask the patient whether she leaks urine on coughing, sneezing or exertion (stress incontinence) or whether she has an urgent need to pass urine before the leakage (urge incontinence). If she gives history of both, she probably has mixed urinary incontinence.
- History of nocturia or frequency with low urinary volume means overactive bladder. This should be managed as for urge incontinence.
- History of previous surgery, and obstetric and gynaecology history may give further clues as to the type of incontinence.
- Amount of leak.
- History of prolapse.
- Severity of symptoms and impact on quality of life (QOL).
- History of constipation.
- Fluid intake (caffeine, alcohol).
- Drug history, e.g. diuretics.
- Social history, e.g. marital status, smoking.
- Family history of incontinence.

Medications that affect continence

These medications may contribute to incontinence:

- sedatives
- diuretics
- anticholinergics
- calcium channel blockers
- antidepressants
- anti-parkinsonian drugs.

Examination

- Height, weight, BMI, waist circumference and blood pressure check.
- Abdominal examination – any palpable mass? This could be palpable bladder, ovarian cyst or a large fibroid.
- Pelvic examination: inspection of the pelvic floor may show visible stress incontinence on straining or coughing. Check for any sign of prolapse, an enlarged uterus on bimanual pelvic examination.
- PR examination if suspicion of constipation or faecal incontinence.
- Neurological examination: if clinically indicated.

Investigations

- Routine urine check for sugar and protein.
- Midstream urine (MSU) for culture and sensitivity to exclude urinary infection.

- Blood glucose: if urine dipstick positive for glucose.
- Urea and electrolytes (U&E) and serum osmolality.
- Bladder diary for three days. Ask the patient to complete a diary of time and fluid volume – intake and output with episodes of urinary leakage, plus her activity at that time. The charts are available from pharmaceutical companies. (Keep the booklets in your examination room.)
- NICE recommends that the use of cystometry, ambulatory urodynamics or videourodynamics is not recommended before starting non-surgical treatment.[8] A reasonable view could be that, for women with genuine stress incontinence (i.e. who leak on activity, coughing or sneezing), without irritative symptoms, who can be shown to leak on clinical examination and who have not undergone a prior procedure for stress incontinence, surgery may be conducted without the need for urodynamic investigation, except a flow rate and a scan. Filling cystometry is used to confirm urodynamic stress incontinence and to exclude detrusor overactivity. Voiding cystometry will demonstrate whether voiding is efficient or whether there is voiding dysfunction.

Suggested urine analysis protocol

In primary care *do not send all urine for MSU.*

- Dipstick urine to detect blood, protein, glucose, leucocytes and nitrites.
- If positive for nitrites and leucocytes and patient has symptoms of urinary tract infection, send for an MSU, treat pending the results. If the patient is asymptomatic treat if MSU is positive.
- If negative for nitrites and leucocytes and patient has symptoms of urinary tract infection, send an MSU. If patient is asymptomatic, no need to send an MSU.

Clinical indications for urodynamic assessment[13]

- Complex mixed urinary symptoms (urge incontinence and stress incontinence).
- Symptoms suggestive of detrusor overactivity unresponsive to pharmacotherapy.
- Voiding dysfunction with incomplete bladder emptying.
- Neuropathic bladder disorder (videourodynamics preferred).

Treatment

The treatment depends on the type of incontinence. Pregnancy and childbirth are known risk factors and there is evidence that pelvic floor exercises during pregnancy reduce risk. The exercises generally are taught during antenatal classes with a midwife.

- For stress incontinence, the first-line therapy is 3 months of pelvic floor exercises. These should be taught by the practice nurse. An instruction leaflet on its own is not enough. There is good evidence that advising pelvic floor exercises is an appropriate treatment for women with persistent postpartum urinary incontinence.[14] *See* Figure 17.1.
- For urge incontinence, bladder training is the first step. The patient should be taught to gradually increase time between voids. *See* Figure 17.2.
- Life style advice in all women with a BMI over 30 kg/m[2].[8]
- Smoking cessation must be advised or a referral to smoking cessation counsellor.
- Management of constipation by diet or laxatives
- Household modifications, mobility aids, downstairs toilets can help an elderly patient struggling to reach the toilet in time.
- Regular prompting of patients to visit the toilet by the residential or nursing home staff can make a lot of difference rather than putting a pad on.
- Patients with overactive bladder should be advised to reduce caffeine, fizzy drinks and alcohol intake.
- Encourage the patient to drink 2 litres of fluid a day. Many women reduce their fluid intake hoping that this will help the symptom control but less fluid intake can lead to concentrated urine which can result in bladder irritation.
- Antimuscarinics are the first-line pharmacological agents used in the treatment of overactive bladder. They have proven to be efficacious and on the whole well tolerated.[15] Oxybutynin is the most widely used antimuscarinic available as an immediate release (IR), extended release (ER) or transdermal patch (TD) preparation. Oxybutynin can be used if bladder training is not successful. NICE recommends that immediate-release oxybutynin should be given as a first line.[8] Transdermal oxybutynin can be given if oral oxybutynin is not tolerated. Compliance is often a problem because of side effects like dryness of mouth, constipation, dry eyes, blurred vision, dizziness and cognitive impairment. Contraindications are acute angle glaucoma, myasthenia gravis, severe ulcerative colitis and GI obstruction.
- NICE does not recommend duloxetine as a first or second line for stress incontinence. It can be considered if there are persisting side effects with oxybutynin.
- Desmopressin or tricyclic antidepressants can be used in women with nocturia.
- Role of HRT is debatable. Although oestrogens may improve atrophic vaginitis, there is no evidence that oestrogens by themselves are beneficial in incontinence.[17]

- Pads and catheters should only be issued on prescription if all treatment options have failed and patient is waiting to see a specialist. These are coping aids.

Follow-up
Telephone consultation is an effective means of follow-up in these patients and can be led by a nurse specialist.[16]

TABLE 17.1 Currently available preparations of antimuscarinic drugs

	ROUTE OF DELIVERY	ADULT DOSAGE
Oxybutynin	Oral Transdermal patch	(a) 2.5–5 mg, 1 to 4 times/day (b) 5–10 mg once daily (SR) One patch, twice/week (3.9 mg/24 hours)
Propiverine	Oral only	15 mg, 2–4 times/day
Solifenacin	Oral only	5–10 mg daily
Tolterodine	Oral only	(a) 1–2 mg, twice daily (b) 4 mg, once daily (SR)
Trospium	Oral only	20 mg, twice daily
Darifenacin	Oral only	7.5 or 15 mg once daily (SR)
Fesoterodine	Oral only	4–8 mg once daily (SR)

SR = sustained release

Source: Price N, Currie I. Urinary incontinence in women: diagnosis and management. *The Practitioner.* March 2010; 254(1727): 27–32. Available at: www.thepractitioner.co.uk

Surgical treatment for stress incontinence
With the advent of minimally invasive surgery and the attraction of day-case surgery, the major procedures like colposuspension have lost their place.

Tension-free vaginal tape (TVT), the new day-case surgical procedure, has become very popular. The procedure produces continence in 80% or more of patients at follow-up of 5 years[18] and NICE has recommended it where non-surgical procedures have not been successful.[19] There are significant benefits in terms of postoperative recovery and return to work.[20]

Pelvic floor muscle training and bladder training[8]
- A trial of supervised pelvic floor muscle training of at least 3 months' duration should be offered as first-line treatment to women with stress or mixed urinary incontinence.
- Pelvic floor training should comprise at least eight contractions performed three times a day.

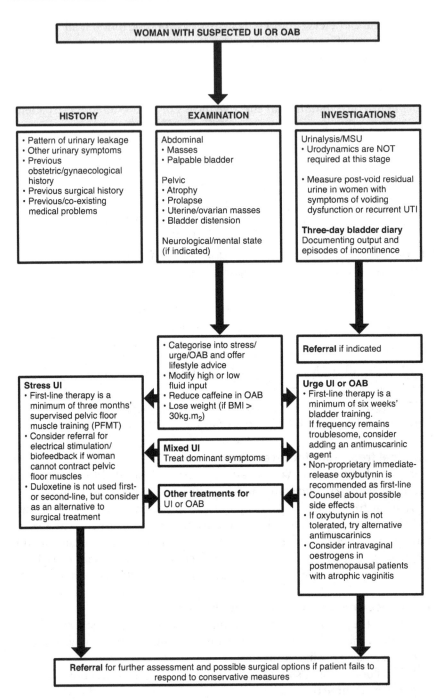

FIGURE 17.1 Summary of pathway for UI[8]

- Electric stimulation should not routinely be used in the treatment of women with overactive bladder.
- If pelvic floor training is beneficial, an exercise programme should be continued.
- Electric stimulation and/or biofeedback should be considered in women who can not actively contract pelvic floor muscles in order to aid motivation and compliance to therapy.

Bladder training should be offered as first-line treatment to women with urge and mixed urinary incontinence for a minimum of six weeks. If no satisfactory response from bladder training programmes, the combination of an antimuscarinic agent with bladder training should be considered if frequency is a troublesome symptom. In women with cognitive impairment and urinary incontinence, prompted and timed voiding programmes are recommended as strategies for reducing leakage episodes.

How to keep a bladder diary
For three consecutive days, record:
- Volume of ALL fluid intake
- Type of drinks
- Measured volume of urine passed on every occasion
- Episodes of urgency
- Time and severity of each incontinence episode

Bladder diary
'Single most useful tool in bladder assesment'. Used for:
- Assessment
- Diagnosis
- Patient education
- Management
- Monitoring progress

FIGURE 17.2 Keeping a bladder diary[8]

Antimuscarinic

Contraindications:
- glaucoma
- ulcerative colitis

- myasthenia gravis
- gastrointestinal obstruction.

Cautions:
- congestive heart failure (CHF)
- coronary heart disease (CHD)
- arrhythmia
- hypothyroidism
- gastro-oesophageal reflux disease (GORD)
- renal impairment.

Side effects:
- dry mouth
- drowsiness
- blurred vision
- constipation
- headaches
- nausea, vomiting
- restlessness
- dry skin
- hot flushes
- palpitations, arrhythmia, tachycardia.

Possible reasons for non-adherence to therapy:
- side effects
- forgetfulness
- purpose of treatment not made clear at the time of issuing the prescription
- not able to afford the prescription cost
- lack of effect.

Referral to secondary care

GPs should refer patients to a urogynaecologist or a surgeon who has experience in this field. Extra contractual referral is not favoured by the Primary Care Trust (try convincing your PCT!).

Urgent referral

An urgent referral should be made for:
- suspected malignant mass
- frank haematuria
- microscopic haematuria in women >50 years

- recurrent or persistent urinary tract infection with haematuria in women >40 years.

Non-urgent referral

A non-urgent referral should be made for:
- prolapse
- palpable bladder
- previous pelvic surgery
- suspected neurological disease
- failure of conservative measures and antimuscarinic drugs.

A referral letter must contain:
- a history of symptoms, duration, severity and impact on quality of life
- examination findings including BMI
- results of investigations if any done
- frequency/volume chart if available
- any treatment so far and benefits/reasons for discontinuation
- patient's expectations.

Practice-based commissioning

An effective community-based service in primary care can reduce unnecessary referrals to hospital and unnecessary follow-ups. A collaboration with a secondary care clinician and the establishment of a local care pathway based on NICE guidelines can provide the right treatment at the right time.

Tariff cost: gynaecology outpatient = £135 (new) and £74 (follow-up).[21]

KEY POINTS

- Urinary incontinence is a common condition which has a significant cost and quality of life impact.
- History alone can often distinguish between the main types of urinary incontinence.
- Abdominal and vaginal examination and urine analysis are recommended at initial consultation.
- A useful tool for diagnosis and management of urinary incontinence is a 3-day bladder diary.
- The NICE guidelines recommend 6 weeks of bladder retraining before considering antimuscarinic therapy, whereas the International Consultation on Incontinence recommends a period of at least 8–12 weeks.
- Oxybutynin is the first-line preparation. All antimuscarinic drugs have a similar level of efficacy.

- Overactive bladder (OAB) is a chronic condition, so regular follow-up is important. This is essential in refractory patients not responding to treatment.
- Pads and catheters should only be used if treatment has failed or as a coping strategy.
- Refer patients with red flag symptoms and if initial treatment is not successful.
- There is a need for improved education for healthcare professionals in the primary care setting about the management of urinary incontinence in women.
- It is important to ensure that before starting medical therapy, patients are counselled and educated about the role of therapy, side effects, and the estimated length of treatment and how long it will take to notice any desired benefits.

Useful websites

For patients – helplines
Bladder and Bowel Foundation: www.bladderandbowelfoundation.org
NHS Choices: www.nhs.uk
www.continence-foundation.org.uk

For GPs
Association for Continence Advice (ACA): www.aca.uk.com
www.nice.org.uk/guidance/CG40

References

1 Hunskaar S, Lose G, Sykes D, *et al.* The prevalence of urinary incontinence in women in four European countries. *BJU International.* 2004; **93**(3): 324–30.
2 Perry S, Shaw C, Assassa P, *et al.* An epidemiological study to establish the prevalence of urinary symptoms and felt need in the community. *J Public Health Med.* 2000; **22**(3): 427–34.
3 Milsom I, Abrams P, Cardozo L, *et al.* How widespread are the symptoms of an overactive bladder and how are they managed? A population based prevalence study. *BJU International.* 2001; **87**(9): 760–6.
4 Landi F, Cesari M, Russo A, *et al.* Potentially reversible risk factors and urinary incontinence in frail older people living in community. *Age Ageing.* 2003; **32**(2): 194–9.
5 Shaw C, Gupta RS, Bushnell DM, *et al.* The extent and severity of urinary incontinence amongst women in UK waiting rooms. *Family Practice.* 2006; **23**(5): 497–506.
6 Sadler C. Combating incontinence after childbirth: conference report. *British Journal of Nursing.* 1996; **5**(7): 448–9.

7 Abrams P, Cardozo L, Fall M, *et al.* The standardisation of terminology of lower urinary tract function: report from the Standard Subcommittee of the International Continence Society. *Neurol Urodyn.* 2002; **21**(2): 167–78.

8 National Institute for Health and Clinical Excellence. Urinary Incontinence: The Management of Urinary Incontinence in Women: NICE guideline 40. London: NIHCE; 2006. www.nice.org.uk/CG040

9 Hannestad YS, Rortveit G, Sandvik H, *et al.* A community-based epidemiological survey of female urinary incontinence. *J Clin Epidemiol.* 2000; **53**(11): 1150–7.

10 Altman D, Granath F, Cnattingius S, *et al.* Hysterectomy and risk of stress urinary incontinence surgery: nationwide cohort study. *Lancet.* 2007; **370**(9597): 1494–9.

11 Prevention and Early Intervention – Continence Services. Feb 2001 www.hscpart nership.org.uk/.../PEI_Learning_Pack_Continence_v9_...

12 Turner DA, Shaw C, McGrother CW, *et al.* The cost of clinically significant urinary symptoms for community dwelling adults in the UK. *BJU Int.* 2004; **93**(9): 1246–53.

13 Price N, Currie I. Urinary incontinence in women: diagnosis and management. *Practitioner.* 2010 Mar; **254**(1727): 27–32. www.thepractitioner.co.uk

14 Hay-Smith J, Mørkved S, Fairbrother KA *et al.* Pelvic floor muscle training for prevention and treatment of urinary and faecal incontinence in antenatal and postnatal women. Cochrane Database Syst Rev. 2008; 4: CD007471.

15 Chapple CR, Khullar V, Gabriel Z, *et al.* The effects of antimuscarinic treatments in overactive bladder: an update of a systematic review and meta-analysis. *Eur Urol.* 2008; **54**(3): 543–62.

16 Jeffery S, Doumouchtsis SK, Fynes M. Patient satisfaction with nurse-led telephone follow-up in women with lower urinary tract symptoms. *J Telemed Telecare.* 2007; **13**(7): 369–73.

17 Shamliyan TA, Kane RL, Wyman J, *et al.* Systematic review: randomised controlled trials of nonsurgical treatments for urinary incontinence in women. *Ann Intern Med.* 2008; **148**(6): 459–73.

18 Rezapour M, Falconer C, Ulmsten U. Tension-free vaginal tape (TVT) in stress incontinence women with intrinsic sphincter deficiency (ISD): a long term follow-up. *Int Urogynecol J Pelvic Floor Dysfunct.* 2001; **12**(Suppl 2): S12–14.

19 National Institute For Clinical Excellence. Final Appraisal Determination Tension-free Vaginal Tape (Gyne-care TVT) for Stress Incontinence. 17 January 2003. Available at: guidance.nice.org.uk >Guidance by type > Appraisals.

20 Ward KL, Hilton P, Browning J. Changes in quality of life following surgery with TVT or colposuspension for primary genuine stress incontinence. *Proc ICS.* 2000. 53: 1150–7.

21 Department of Health. Payment by results. 20 September 2012. Available at: www. dh.gov.uk/paymentbyresults (accessed 15 December 2012).

18

Urinary retention: a primary care emergency

DEFINITION

Acute urinary retention is defined as a sudden inability to pass urine. It can be associated with abdominal pain or can be painless.

Chronic urinary retention is defined as long-standing incomplete voiding of the bladder.

From a primary care physician perspective both the conditions require immediate admission.

Causes

Urinary retention may be caused by:

- constipation
- recurrent urinary tract infections
- urethral strictures/calculus
- spinal cord compression
- disc prolapse
- anticholinergics
- tricyclic antidepressants
- Parkinson's disease
- postoperative pelvic surgery
- idiopathic detrusor failure
- postmenopausal women due to oestrogen deficiency (rare)
- Fowler's syndrome: electromyographic (EMG) abnormality of the striated urethral sphincter.[1]

Primary care management
History
Enquire about the history of:
- the duration of sudden inability to pass urine
- abdominal pain
- recurrent urinary tract infections, constipation
- haematuria or passing clots
- taking drugs: anticholinergics, tricyclic antidepressants, antihistamines.

Examination
Per abdominal examination:
- an enlarged tender bladder
- neurological examination is only necessary if suspecting a neurological cause
- Per rectal (PR) examination to exclude constipation.

Investigations
Investigations should include:
- urine analysis
- kidney function tests (U&E) to exclude renal impairment
- ultrasound scan of abdomen and pelvis.

There is no point doing these tests in primary care as they will be carried out in the hospital.

Management
- Acute retention requires urgent catheterisation and further investigations.
- Catheterisation is not always necessary in patients with chronic retention. These patients require a referral to a urologist.
- Constipation management as per NICE guidelines. See below.

NICE guidelines on the diagnosis and management of constipation[2]
Definitions:
- **Chronic constipation**: if lasting longer than 8 weeks.
- **Idiopathic constipation**: if unexplained by any anatomical, physiological, radiological or histological abnormalities.
- **Intractable constipation**: if not responding to sustained optimum medical management.

History:
- Stool pattern: fewer than three complete stools per week

- — overflow soiling
- — large infrequent stools
- — rabbit droppings.
- Associated symptoms:
  - — poor appetite
  - — abdominal pains
  - — straining
  - — anal pain.
- Past history:
  - — anal fissure
  - — constipation
  - — bleeding.
- Digital rectal examination (DRE): ensure privacy, informed consent and presence of chaperone.

Management:
- advice on balanced diet and fluid intake
- disimpaction – oral/rectal
- maintenance therapy.

Ongoing support:
- provide tailored follow-up
- refer patient if no response to treatment within 3 months.

KEY POINTS

- Acute urinary retention is defined as a sudden inability to pass urine with symptoms of an enlarged tender bladder.
- In chronic retention many patients are asymptomatic.
- All cases of retention must be referred to secondary care as an emergency.

References

1 Kavia RB, Datta SN, Dasgupta R, *et al.* Urinary retention in women: its causes and management. *BJU Int.* 2006; **97**(2): 281–7.
2 National Collaborating Centre for Women's and Children's Health. Constipation in Children and Young People: Diagnosis and Management of Idiopathic Childhood Constipation in Primary and Secondary Care: NICE guideline 99. London: RCOG Press; 2010. (Commissioned by National Institute for Health and Clinical Excellence.) http://publications.nice.org.uk/constipation-in-children-and-young-people-cg99

19

Endometriosis

Endometriosis is one of the most common gynaecological diseases and a common cause of chronic pelvic pain in women of reproductive age.

DEFINITION

Endometriosis is a condition defined as the presence of functional endometrial glandular and stromal tissue at various extrauterine sites. This induces a chronic inflammatory reaction resulting in the formation of scar tissue. Extrauterine endometrial tissue can occur anywhere in the body but the most common sites are the pelvis, peritoneum and bowel. Less common sites are the lungs and brain.

The endometrial tissue deposits may be small or large, causing significant morbidity such as endometriotic cysts that affect the ovaries.

Prevalence

It is rather difficult to determine the prevalence due to the difficulty in diagnosis because of the variable nature of endometriosis, and its severity and diversity of symptoms. It is estimated to affect 5%–10% of women in the reproductive age group.[1] It mainly affects fertile women and is more common in those who reach early menarche or a late menopause. Its prevalence in sub-fertile women is estimated to be between 25%–40%.[2]

Aetiology

The aetiology is not fully understood. Retrograde menstruation theory explains the pelvic disease. The distant endometrial deposits are thought to be due to immunological and embryological factors.

Risk factors

Risk factors include:

- obstruction of menstrual outflow (mullerian anomalies)
- short menstrual cycle
- low birth weight
- exposure to endocrine-disrupting chemicals[19]
- prolonged exposure to endogenous oestrogens, obesity, late menopause, early menarche.

Primary care management

Endometriosis is often labelled as 'missed disease'. On average it takes about 7–8 years to reach a diagnosis.[3] The delay is usually due to failure in diagnosis. The condition may be asymptomatic, causing mild symptoms or may be debilitating, affecting the patient's quality of life (QOL).[4]

History

Cyclical bleeding from ectopic endometrial tissue causing inflammation, scarring and adhesions explains the pathogenesis of the symptoms.[5] The presentation of symptoms is variable and may include the following:[6,7]

- dysmenorrhoea
- deep dyspareunia
- difficult or painful defecation
- dyschezia
- chronic pelvic pain: *this can cause depression, sexual dysfunction and relationship disharmony*[8]
- low back pain
- painful micturition
- bloating
- menorrhagia
- infertility
- haematuria
- haemoptysis
- diarrhoea
- cyclical rectal bleed
- seizures
- lethargy.

Pelvic examination

A pelvic examination must be carried out in all patients presenting with dysmenorrhoea, deep pelvic pain, dyspareunia and painful defecation.

- Pelvic examination may be essentially normal; this does not rule out endometriosis.
- Pelvic and uterosacral ligament tenderness and fixed retroverted uterus are most common positive findings.
- Palpable deep infiltrating nodules either in the pouch of Douglas or uterosacral ligaments are more confirmatory findings as per guidelines. These nodules are easily demonstrable during menstruation and may be occasionally visible in the vagina or on the cervix. There is, however, evidence that performing the examination during menstruation helps to make the diagnosis, but many women will be reluctant to be examined at this time.[26]
- Bowel or bladder symptoms in some patients make the diagnosis difficult to distinguish from irritable bowel syndrome or interstitial cystitis.[26]

Investigations

- The gold-standard diagnostic test is laparoscopy with lesion biopsy[9] but the absence of visible endometriosis does not equate to the absence of the condition, because its accuracy depends on the expertise of the clinician performing the laparoscopy and the timing of the procedure in relation to menstruation.
- Serum CA125 has been used to help in diagnosis but it is non-specific so not reliable.[28]
- Ultrasound: transvaginal ultrasound (TVS) has been shown to be a highly sensitive tool for detection of ovarian endometriosis. A recent systemic review showed that TVS is an accurate test for non-invasive detection of deep infiltrating endometriosis of the recto sigmoid.[10]
- Magnetic resonance imaging (MRI) is of limited value in diagnosing any peritoneal disease.
- Biochemical markers: a recent study showed that women with endometriosis have higher levels of IL-10,1 FN-gamma and IL-4, showing a shift towards increased inflammatory cytokines.[11]

Treatment

The Royal College of Obstetricians and Gynaecologists (RCOG) suggests it is reasonable to treat the patient empirically.[9]

The management of endometriosis can be medical or surgical. None of the options have been shown to reduce the recurrence of symptoms once the treatment is stopped.

Factors affecting treatment choices:

- age
- previous treatment

- severity of pain
- fertility status
- resources and cost
- patient's attitude.

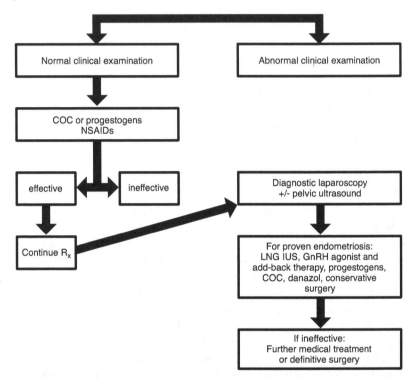

FIGURE 19.1 Management of endometriosis with pain
Source: www.prescriber.co.uk

Medical treatment

Eighty to ninety per cent of patients can have symptomatic benefits with medical treatment.

1. Analgesia for pain control: analgesia should be the first line of treatment in younger patients and also those waiting for the confirmation of diagnosis. This could be a challenge for the GP who must balance the effectiveness of treatment against the tolerability and the risk of adverse side effects. Non-NSAID agents (paracetamol, codeine and dihydrocodeine) are good baseline analgesics and are well tolerated. Remember the liver toxicity in overdose; should be used with caution in patients with alcoholic liver disease, hepatic or renal impairment. Ibuprofen or naproxen are the traditional first-line NSAID agents. Variable patient

tolerance, gastrointestinal side effects, possible increased risk of cardio-vascular events with long-term, high dose use and four-times-a-day dose are the possible drawbacks. There is no good evidence supporting the efficacy of NSAIDs.

2. Acupuncture may effectively reduce the pain of endometriosis but supporting evidence is limited. The conclusion is based on a Cochrane review of randomised single- or double-blind controlled trials of women with laparoscopically confirmed diagnosis of endometriosis.[24]

3. Endometrial tissue is oestrogen dependent and suppressing oestrogen production is the aim of medical management. Suppression of ovarian function for at least 6 months is the basis for hormonal treatment and the options could be combined hormonal treatment (COC), progesterone-only hormonal contraceptive pill (POP) and gonadotrophin-releasing hormone agonists.[12]

Medical treatment has been used in combination with surgical treatment to improve response. Pre-surgical treatment makes surgery safer and easier and post-surgical treatment treats areas that escape resection. Patients must be fully informed in the decision making where hormonal management is prescribed pre- or post-surgical intervention.

COCs are effective for pain control and taken in a tricyclic regimen can reduce menstrual blood loss. COCs are effective maintenance therapy post-surgery and for patients not wishing to conceive. Nausea, headaches and weight gain are the common side effects. Past history of migraine, hypertension and thrombo-embolism are the absolute contraindications of COCs. Irregular menstrual bleeding, fluid retention, bloating and breast tenderness can limit the use of progestogens but they can be effective for pain relief.

TABLE 19.1 Common side effects of drug treatment

DRUG TREATMENT	COMMON SIDE EFFECTS
NSAIDs: ibuprofen, mefenamic acid	Abdominal side effects
Combined oral contraceptives (COCs)	Headaches/migraines, increased risk of thromboembolism
Progestogens (POP)	Fluid retention, bloating and breast tenderness
Danazol	Androgenic: acne, weight gain

4. Intrauterine coil: the levonorgestrel intrauterine system (LNG-IUS; Mirena coil) has been shown to reduce pain. It works by releasing a low and steady level of levonorgestrel progestogen. In a small uncontrolled trial, the LNG-IUS seemed to control symptoms in mild to moderate

endometriosis even after 3 years of use, although the discontinuation rate of coil was high.[13] A systematic review in 2010 showed that the LNG-IUS reduces the recurrence of painful periods in women who have had surgical treatment of endometriosis as compared to the control group.[14]

5. Gonadotrophin-releasing hormone agonists (GnRH agonists): these are usually administered monthly in depot injection form. They produce an initial stimulatory response followed by down-regulation of follicle stimulating hormone (FSH) and lutenising hormone (LH), resulting in suppression of ovarian steroidogenesis. GnRH is a peptide hormone produced by the hypothalamus that stimulates the anterior lobe of the pituitary gland to make follicle stimulating hormones (FSHs) and luteinising hormones (LHs). The most common is Zoladex, used as a subcutaneous injection 3.6 mg every 28 days; maximum duration of treatment 6 months. It is effective and the benefit lasts for a few months post treatment. However there is a high recurrence rate: one study found 53% after 2 years.[15] The most common side effects are related to inhibition of oestrogen production. Hot flushes, increased sweating, vaginal dryness, dyspareunia, loss of libido and loss of bone mineral density are the common side effects. These can be alleviated by giving a low-dose oestrogen in the form of hormone replacement therapy, tibolone or low-dose continuous combined hormone replacement therapy (HRT) to prevent endometrial hyperplasia if treatment is needed for more than a few weeks.

   No significant difference in terms of dysmenorrhoea control was observed in women treated with COCs or those treated with GnRH at 6 months' follow-up after discontinuing treatment (or 0.48; 95% CI 0.08–2.90).[16]

6. Danazol: works by inhibiting pituitary gonadotrophins; it combines androgenic activity with antioestrogenic and antiprogestogenic activity. Nausea, dizziness, weight gain, vaginal dryness, reduction in breast size, hair loss, acne, oily skin, voice change and hirsutism are common androgenic side effects which outweigh the benefits. A rare side effect of clitoral hypertrophy is unacceptable to women. The recommended dose in endometriosis is 200–800 mg daily in divided doses adjusted to achieve amenorrhoea, usually for 3–6 months.

7. Aromatase inhibitors: these work by blocking the enzyme aromatase cytochrome P-459 which converts androgens into oestrogens. Decreasing the production of oestrogens is the principle behind their use. They are used in treatment of breast cancer and ovarian cancer in postmenopausal women. The use of aromatase inhibitors in endometriosis management is unlicensed. Only one RCT showed that the combination of a GnRH

agonist and aromatase inhibitor is more effective than a GnRH agonist alone in improving pain in the postoperative period.[17]

8. Long-chain omega-3 fatty acids: the latest results from the Nurses' Health Study (a long-term epidemiological study) suggest that omega-3 fatty acids may reduce the risk of endometriosis. During the 12-year study, it was found that women consuming the high intake of long-chain omega-3 fatty acids were 22% less likely to be diagnosed with endometriosis.[27]

Surgical treatment

The success of the surgery depends on the disease severity and its location. The ideal surgical treatment would be to remove all visible endometriosis, although this is not always possible. Surgical options are ablation, excisional surgery if ovarian endometrioma, adhesiolysis and total abdominal hysterectomy with bilateral salpingo-oophorectomy.

1. Ablation: ablation with carbon dioxide (CO_2), bipolar diathermy, unipolar diathermy or helium thermal coagulator are all popular methods. Ablation of lesions has been shown to reduce endometriosis-related pain compared to diagnostic laparoscopy only.[29] Laparoscopic uterine nerve ablation was thought to improve pain, however a Cochrane review showed this is ineffective.[30] Removing entire lesions in severe and deeply infiltrating disease significantly improves pain.[28]

2. Excisional surgery: the risk of trauma to adjacent tissue and the postoperative adhesions are the main disadvantages of excisional surgery. The only indication of this form of treatment is in patients with ovarian endometrioma to avoid the risk of recurrence. Excision of endometriotic deposits is also advocated in pelvic peritoneal disease.

3. Total abdominal hysterectomy with bilateral salpingo-oophorectomy (TAH with BSO). This major operation is only indicated in patients with advanced endometriosis. Patients undergoing TAH alone should be counselled about the possibility of persisting symptoms after the operation.[28]

Endometriosis after hysterectomy

There is very little evidence to suggest that endometriosis may be reactivated in women following a hysterectomy with bilateral salpingo-oophorectomy (TAH &BSO) who start hormone replacement therapy (HRT). As a precautionary measure, long-term low dose oestrogen replacement therapy or tibolone is required in these patients.[18]

Endometriosis and ovarian cancer

A recent US study, by University of Southern California researchers, found women with endometriosis were at greater risk of three forms of ovarian cancer. A history of endometriosis was reported by 20.2% of women with clear cells, 13.9% with endometrioid and 9.2% with low-grade serous subtypes of invasive ovarian cancer. A history of endometriosis was not associated with a risk of mucinous or high-grade serous invasive ovarian cancer. Ovarian surgery was found to reduce the risk of cancer linked to endometriosis.[20]

The consensus view is that although endometriosis increases the relative risk of developing cancer, absolute risk remains low.

Endometriosis and infertility

Endometriotic implants are associated with an inflammatory process. This results in the formation of adhesions thus interfering with ovarian and tubal function. Pain due to endometriosis can reduce the frequency of sexual intercourse, ovarian adhesions can inhibit the release of oocytes, ovarian endometriosis can affect ovarian function and formation of adhesions can affect tubal peristalsis. More recent evidence suggests that pelvic endometriosis may interfere with implantation and may be the pathway through which endometriosis impairs fertility.[21]

Overall, about half the women with endometriosis will suffer from infertility and about half the infertile women will have endometriosis. A randomised controlled trial (RCT) has shown that operative laparoscopy for early stage endometriosis improves fertility.[22] Diagnosing and treating endometriosis in women with previous in vitro fertilisation (IVF) failure will increase the chance of both IVF and natural conception success.[23]

Chinese herbal medicine for endometriosis

In China, treatment of endometriosis using Chinese herbal medicine is routine.[25] Chinese randomised controlled trials (RCTs) involving 158 women were included. Both trials described adequate methodology and neither trial compared Chinese herbal medicine with placebo treatment. Post-surgical administration of Chinese herbal medicine may have comparable benefits to gestrinone but with fewer side effects. Oral Chinese herbal medicine may have a better overall treatment effect than danazol and may be more effective in dysmenorrhoea and shrinkage of adnexal masses when used in conjunction with Chinese herbal enema. However more vigorous research is required to assess the role of Chinese herbal medications in the treatment of endometriosis.[25]

KEY POINTS

- Endometriosis is a common condition affecting women of reproductive age.
- Endometriosis may be asymptomatic or debilitating and has a profound effect on quality of life.
- The pain of endometriosis can significantly affect women's quality of life. It is important to provide good and effective analgesia.
- The gold standard test is laparoscopy.
- Endometriosis can be managed either medically or surgically.
- COCs, progestogens and GnRH analogues relieve endometrial-associated pain equally well.
- Refer the patient if there is no response to medical treatment, but consider the possibility of an alternative diagnosis.
- Surgical ablation of endometrial lesions is the definitive treatment.
- There is no role of medical management in the treatment of endometriosis-associated infertility.
- Endometriosis can triple the risk of ovarian cancer but absolute risk remains low.

Useful websites

For GPs

Royal College of Obstetricians and Gynaecologists. Endometriosis: investigation and management. Green-top guideline 24. RCOG; 2006. www.rcog.org.uk/womens-health/clinical-guidance/investigation-and-management-endometriosis-green-top-24

References

1 Winkel CA. Evaluation and management of women with endometriosis. *Obstet Gynaecol.* 2003; **102**(2): 397–408.

2 Ozkan S, Murk W, Arici A. Endometriosis and infertility: epidemiology and evidence-based treatments. *Ann N Y Acad Sci.* 2008; 1127: 92–100.

3 Endometriosis | BMJ. Endometriosis still takes 8 years to diagnose and treatment options remain largely ineffective. Press release. 15 September 2005. Available at: www.bmj.com/content/340bmj.c2168?ijkey=LFjvs2BsftdQo

4 Farquhar C. Clinical review: endometriosis. *BMJ.* 2007; 334: 249–53.

5 Nawathe A, Patwardhan S, Yates D, *et al.* Systematic review of the effects of aromatase inhibitors on pain associated with endometriosis. *BJOG.* 2008; **115**(7): 818–22.

6 Louden SF, Wingfield M, Read PA, *et al.* The incidence of atypical symptoms in patients with endometriosis. *J Obstet Gynaecol.* 1995; 15: 307–10.

7 Meurs-Szojda MM, Mijatovic V, Felt-Bersma RJF, *et al.* Irritable bowel syndrome

and chronic constipation in patients with endometriosis. *Colorectal Dis.* 2011; **13**(1): 67–71.

8 Ballard KD, Seaman HE, de Vries CS, *et al.* Can symptomatology help in the diagnosis of endometriosis? Findings from a national case-control study: part 1. *BJOG.* 2008; 115(11): 1382–91.

9 Kennedy S, Bergqvist A, Chapron C. ESHRE guideline for the diagnosis and treatment of endometriosis. *Hum Reprod.* 2005; **20**(10): 2698–704. Available online at: http://Humrep.oxfordjournals.org/content/20/10/2698.full

10 Hudelist G, English J, Thomas AE, *et al.* Diagnostic accuracy of transvaginal ultrasound for non-invasive diagnosis of bowel endometriosis: systematic review and meta-analysis. *Ultrasound Obstet Gynecol.* 2011; **37**(3): 257–63.

11 Podgaec S, Abrão MS, Dias Jr JA, *et al.* Endometriosis: an inflammatory disease with a Th2 immune response component. *Hum Reprod.* 2007; **22**(5): 1373–9.

12 Kennedy S, Bergqvist A, Chapron C, *et al.* EHSRE guidelines for the diagnosis and treatment of endometriosis. *Hum Rep.* 2005; 20: 2698–704.

13 Lockhat FB, Emembolu JO, Konje JC. The efficacy, side-effects and continuation rates in women with symptomatic endometriosis undergoing treatment with an intra-uterine administered progestogen (levonorgestrel): a 3 year follow-up. *Hum Reprod.* 2005; **20**(3): 789–93.

14 Abou-Setta AM, Al-Inany HG, Farquhar CM. Levonorgestrel-releasing intrauterine device (LNG-IUD) for symptomatic endometriosis following surgery. Cochrane Database Syst Rev. 2006; **18**(4): CD005072.

15 Walker K, Shaw R. Gonadotrophin-releasing hormone analogues for the treatment of endometriosis: long term follow up. *Fertil Steril.* 1993; 59: 511–15.

16 Davis L, Kennedy SS, Moore J *et al.* Modern combined oral contraceptive for pain associated with endometriosis. Cochrane Database Syst Rev. 2007; 18(3); CD001019.

17 Soysal S, Soysal ME, Ozer S, *et al.* The effects of post surgical administration of goserelin plus anastrozole compared to goserelin alone in patients with severe endometriosis: a prospective randomised trial. *Hum Reprod.* 2004; **19**(1): 160–7.

18 Soliman NF, Hillard TC. Hormone replacement therapy in women with past history of endometriosis. *Climacteric.* 2006; **9**(5): 325–35.

19 Giudice LS. Clinical practice. Endometriosis. *N Engl J Med.* 2010; **362**(25); 2389–98.

20 Association between endometriosis and risk of histological subtypes of ovarian cancer. *Lancet Oncol.* [online] 22 February 2012. Available online at: www.thelancet.com/journal/lanonc/PIIS1470-2045(11)70404-1

21 Lessey B, Castelbaum A, Sawin S, *et al.* Aberrant integrin expression in the endometrium of women with endometriosis. *J Clin Endocrinol Metab.* 1994; 79: 643–9.

22 Marcoux S, Maheux R, Berube S. Laparoscopic surgery in infertile women with minimal or mild endometriosis. *N Engl J Med.* 1997; 337: 217–22.

23 Littman E, Giudice L, Lathi R, *et al.* Role of laparoscopic treatment of endometriosis in patients with failed in vitro fertilisation cycles. *Fertil Steril.* 2005; 84: 1574–8.

24 Zhu X, Hamilton KD, McNicol ED. Acupuncture for pain in endometriosis. Cochrane Database Syst Rev. 2011; 9: CD007864.

25 Flower A, Liu JP, Chen S, *et al.* Chinese herbal medicine for endometriosis. Cochrane Database Syst Rev, 2009; 3: CD006568.

26 Wills H, Demetriou C, May K, *et al.* NHS evidence: women's health – annual evidence update on endometriosis – clinical features and diagnosis. Oxford: Nuffield Department of Obstetrics and Gynaecology; 2010. Available at: www.library.nhs.uk//womenshealth/ViewResource.aspx?resID=307263 (accessed 15 December 2012).

27 Missmer SA, Chavarro JE, Malspeis S. A prospective study of dietary fat consumption and endometriosis risk. *Hum Reprod.* 2010; **25**(6): 1528–35.

28 Royal College of Obstetricians and Gynaecologists. Endometriosis: investigation and management. Green-top guideline 24. RCOG; 2006.

29 Sutton CJG, Ewen SP, Whitelaw N, *et al.* Prospective, randomised double-blinded, controlled trial of laser laparoscopy in the treatment of pelvic pain associated with minimal, mild and moderate endometriosis. *Fertil Steril.* 1994; 62: 696–700.

30 Proctor M, Latthe P, Farquhar C, *et al.* Surgical interruption of pelvic nerve pathways for primary and secondary dysmenorrhoea. Cochrane Database Syst Rev. 2005; 4: CD001896.

20

Menopause

DEFINITION

Menopause or change of life is a normal physiological process, not an illness. It is a retrospective diagnosis, 12 months after periods have stopped.

The average age of menopause in Western women is 51.5 years, however there is a wide range extending from the 30s to the 60s. It is often earlier in less well-developed countries and in smokers. It is suggested that the onset of menopause may be associated with less energy expenditure and fat oxidation.

Perimenopause

A period of two or three years before a woman's period finally stops is defined as perimenopause. A menstrual irregularity of frequent cycles followed by less frequent longer cycles and finally stopping of bleeding is the usual menopause transition.

Premature menopause

The British Menopause Society (BMS) defines premature menopause as cessation of menstrual bleeding under the age of 45 years.[1] Premature menopause affects an estimated 1% of women below the age of 40 years and 0.1% below the age of 30 years. It is a common condition and is responsible for 4%–18% of cases of secondary amenorrhoea and 10%–28% of primary amenorrhoea.[2] Mean life expectancy in women with premature menopause below the age of 40 years is on average 2 years less than that in women with menopause after the age of 55 years.[3]

Aetiology of premature menopause

Primary:

- chromosomal: Turner's syndrome, Down's syndrome
- metabolic: galactosaemia
- disruption of oestrogen synthesis
- abnormality of follicle stimulating hormone (FSH) receptor.

Secondary:

- surgical: bilateral oophorectomy; hysterectomy without bilateral oophorectomy can induce ovarian failure
- radiotherapy
- chemotherapy
- infection (rarely), mumps, tuberculosis.

Causes

Menopause results from loss of ovarian follicular function due to ageing. Other causes:

- radiotherapy
- chemotherapy
- surgery.

Symptoms

The symptoms vary widely. A majority of women experience no symptoms while some may suffer from debilitating symptoms. Symptoms are attributed to tissue sensitivity to lower levels of oestrogen. Some women become symptomatic while still having periods. The symptoms depend on genetic, ethnic, cultural, educational, economic, environmental, family and lifestyle factors. In the Study of Women's Health Across the Nation (SWAN), significantly more African American and Hispanic and fewer Chinese and Japanese than Caucasian women reported vasomotor symptoms. Fewer vasomotor symptoms were reported by women with postgraduate education.[4] The common symptoms are outlined below.

Vasomotor:

- Hot flushes. Recent epidemiological studies suggest that overweight women have 1.5–2 times increased risk of hot flushes and this risk increases with severity of obesity.[5] Some studies have found that subcutaneous adiposity is most related to hot flushes. Hot flushes can occur at any time of the day and night, and can disturb normal sleep patterns.
- Night sweats.[6]

- Palpitations.
- Poor sleep.[6]
- Irritability.[6]
- Loss of concentration.[6]
- Poor memory making more mistakes.[6]
- Emotional lability and tearfulness.

Urogenital:
- Dry vagina.
- Vaginal itching. It is the lack of oestrogens that causes vaginal dryness resulting in vaginal itching.
- Dyspareunia.
- Poor sex drive causing relationship problems.
- Cystocele, rectocele and uterine prolapse. Being obese or overweight is associated with progression in cystocele, rectocele and uterine prolapse.[7]
- Ovarian cysts are common in postmenopausal women.[8,9] The incidence has been reported variably between 1% and 13% in postmenopausal women and up to 49% in premenopausal women treated with tamoxifen.[10]
- Urinary frequency, urgency or bladder irritability.[1]
- Urinary incontinence due to prolapse which is increased by obesity
- Frequent urinary infections.

Others:
- Bony aches and pains especially lumbar spine and hips due to osteoporosis. Half of postmenopausal women will suffer a fracture during their lifetime, mainly because of osteoporosis.
- Weight gain.
- Metabolic syndrome. Higher waist circumference, BMI, triglycerides, blood sugar and HDL-cholesterol.
- Increased risk of coronary heart disease (CHD).
- Venous thromboembolism (VTE). Obesity and hormone replacement therapy increase the risk of VTE. Increased BMI and transdermal oestrogen users had similar risk as increased BMI and non-users.[11]

Primary care management

History
- Duration of symptoms and trial of any over-the-counter medications.
- Associated urinary symptoms.
- Sexual history.

- Family history of early menopause.
- Past history of surgery, chemotherapy or radiotherapy.

Examination

This will not be necessary in a majority of women.

- Inspection of vulva to exclude any vulval or vaginal pathology.
- Bimanual pelvic examination if history of heavy/irregular bleed.
- Look and examine for prolapse (*see* Chapter 14).
- Per speculum examination to exclude cervical polyp or erosion.
- Vaginal swabs or smear test if indicated.

Investigations

- Height, weight, BMI, waist circumference, blood pressure check and pulse check. Using both BMI and waist circumference to assess risk of cardiovascular disease and diabetes, 14%, 16% and 23% are at increased risk, at high risk and at very high risk respectively.[12]
- If raised blood pressure, checking of fasting cholesterol, fasting blood sugar and calculate JBS score. Obesity is a significant risk factor for cardiovascular disease.
- Full blood count (FBC) if heavy or frequent bleeding.
- Serum follicle-stimulating hormone (FSH). It is unnecessary to check FSH in women over the age of 45 years as every woman over this age is perimenopausal. The only indications of measuring FSH are in a young woman after total abdominal hysterectomy with conservation of ovaries with vasomotor or urogenital symptoms or in a woman with a history of premature menopause. Two FSH tests taken 4–6 weeks apart with a reading of >30 IU/L indicates sustained ovarian responsiveness.
- Autoimmune screen for multiple endocrine conditions.
- Chromosome analysis in women below the age of 30 years.
- ACTH stimulation test if Addison's disease is suspected.
- The Fracture Risk Assessment Tool (FRAX) can be used to calculate a patient's 10-year absolute risk of fracture.
- DEXA scan screening to exclude osteoporosis. Both age and oestradiol deficiency can cause changes on the bone density in the lumbar spine, femoral neck and trochanter. The diagnosis is made when bone mineral density (BMD) on dual X-ray absorptiometry (DXA) is 2.5 standard deviation (SD) below the young adult mean (T score < −2.5).

Treatment

The menopause is associated with osteoporosis and development of risk factors for cardiovascular disease. The risk factors for cardiovascular disease include adverse effect on lipid profile and impaired glucose metabolism.

Women's risk of death from ischaemic heart disease (IHD) does not rise sharply at menopause. It increases gradually with age. Researchers used age and sex-specific mortality from England, Wales and the US between 1950 and 2000 for three birth cohorts: 1916–25, 1926–35 and 1936–45 and concluded that gender differences in risk is because of the acceleration in men's risk of dying at younger age group with ischaemic heart disease rather than protective effects of women's premenopausal hormones.[13]

- Health promotional advise regarding weight, stopping smoking, reducing alcohol intake and increasing exercise to at least three times a week for half an hour.
- Weight gain prevention should be recognised as an important goal for women before they reach menopause.
- Referral to a commercial weight loss organisation is more effective than standard primary care treatment in helping obese and overweight women. Researchers in a controlled study in the UK, Germany and Australia randomised 722 obese and overweight patients to 12 months' standard care or to 12 months' free membership of Weight Watchers and found that weight loss was significantly greater in the Weight Watchers group, with a mean loss from baseline of 5.06 kg as compared to 2.25 kg for those receiving standard care.[14]
- Elevated blood pressure, lipid levels and diabetes must be managed as per NICE guidelines.[15,16,17,18]
- Encourage reducing caffeine, and cutting down on spicy food and alcohol as they may relieve menopausal hot flushes.
- Exercise: the evidence suggests that exercise has a small statistically significant effect on bone mineral density. This finding comes from a meta-analysis of randomised controlled studies by Cochrane researchers.[19] Exercise also improves cardiovascular risk and should be part of a healthy lifestyle for all women. Non-weight bearing, high-force exercise such as progressive resistance strength training in the lower limbs, had the greater benefit for bone mineral density (BMD) at the hip. The most effective exercise for BMD at the spine was a combination exercise programme.
- Denosumab (Prolia) has been recommended by the Scottish Medicines Consortium (SMC) for the prevention of osteoporotic fractures in postmenopausal women. Women should have a bone mineral density (BMD) T-score of between < −2.5 and ≥ −4.0, and be unable to take oral bisphosphonates because of contraindications, intolerance or inability to comply with administration instructions. The SMC's recommendation follows guidance issued 2 months earlier by NICE (http://guidance.nice.uk/TA204). To be eligible for denosumab under NICE guidance, women must have a combination of age, clinical risk

factors and T-score that are likely to restrict the treatment to women in England who are at highest risk.

- Herbal products: herbal medicines for menopausal symptoms are very popular and a majority are over-the-counter. The most common reason for trying these products over the counter was a perceived risk of side effects with hormone replacement therapy.[20] The evidence base for using herbal products remains poor. Black cohosh (*Cimicifuga racemosa L. Nutt*) is the most commonly used herbal medicine for relief of hot flushes and sweats. A recent review of randomised controlled trials (RCTs) failed to find evidence for the clinical effectiveness of black cohosh at a dose of 40 mg.[21] A number of recent case reports have linked black cohosh with acute liver disease.[22] Reports of hepatotoxicity, in some cases requiring transplantation, prompted the Medicines and Healthcare Products Regulatory Agency (MHRA) to recommend that warnings be added to products containing black cohosh (www.ukmi.nhs.uk).

  St John's wort, dose of 900 mg taken daily for 3 months, has been found to have a beneficial effect on psychological symptoms of the menopause in one controlled study.[23] Two placebo-controlled double blind RCTs showed combination of black cohosh and St John's wort beneficial in both climacteric and psychological symptoms and a positive effect on lipid metabolism.[24] The dose used in one of the large trial was 0.25 mg of St John's wort extract and two tablets orally twice daily for 8 weeks followed by one tablet twice a day for the next 8 weeks.[24]

  Red clover may show some benefit for relieving vasomotor symptoms because it contains phytooestrogens. Evening primrose oil, *Ginko biloba*, ginseng, sage, lemon balm, wild yam, flax seed and liquorice root are some of the popular herbal medicines with little or no evidence of benefit.

- Non-hormonal: there are several non-hormonal options for the management of vasomotor symptoms. Evidence suggests that SSRIs such as fluoxetine and SNRIs such as venlafaxine may reduce hot flushes. Gabapentin has also been shown to improve hot flushes compared with placebo.

Hormone replacement therapy (HRT)

Since the publications of Women's Health Initiative (WHI) studies, the understanding of HRT has improved a great deal. It is clear that the use of age-appropriate doses can help to improve symptoms while minimising the risks.[25] HRT is now recommended for the short-term treatment of vasomotor symptoms such as hot flushes. But hot flushes may return even if HRT is withdrawn gradually. The study included 81 postmenopausal women using HRT to manage hot flushes, who were randomised to either gradual withdrawal or abrupt discontinuation of treatment. By the end of the year, approximately 1 in every 2 women had restarted HRT.[26] It is therefore important to provide women with practical advice on how to manage symptoms if they decide to discontinue treatment.

Oestrogen replacement remains the most effective treatment to reduce symptoms. The MHRA advice, based on data from the WHI and the Million Women Study stated that hormone replacement therapy may be used for severe menopausal symptoms if the woman understands the side effects.[27,28,29] It also stated that the replacement therapy should be prescribed in the lowest possible dose for the shortest period of time. This, of course, does not apply to those with premature ovarian failure who should be encouraged to take HRT until they are 50. There is no fixed time when risks outweigh benefits and each woman must be assessed and treated on an individual basis. Some women may need a longer therapy.

Women with an intact uterus will need a sequential preparation of HRT, containing continuous oestrogen and 12 days of progestogen, if they are within 12 months of their menopause. Those who have passed 12 months since last menstrual bleed can take a continuous combined preparation. These preparations are not totally bleed-free and about 50% of women can expect some bleeding in the first year of use. Heavier bleeding must be investigated. A levonorgestrel IUS could be a good alternative. This gives good endometrial protection and oestrogen alone can be given for replacement.

Tibolone with oestrogenic, progestogenic and weak androgenic activity can be used for treatment of vasomotor symptoms and osteoporosis prophylaxis. There is evidence that it improves libido.[30]

After a hysterectomy the only requirement is oestrogen replacement, unless there is pre-existing endometriosis – in which case a continuous combined form should be used.

In the last few years there has been a huge amount of adverse publicity linking HRT with increased risk of developing breast cancer. The Women's Health Initiative (WHI) study, in which women took continuous combined HRT, showed an increased risk of developing breast cancer (0.8/1000 per year), or four extra cases for every five years of therapy per 1000 women. This is against a background of 45 women per 1000 between the ages of 50 and 70 years.[28]

Paradoxically, the study showed no increase in the incidence of breast cancer in women on oestrogen-only preparations.[28] Therefore it is essential to counsel and involve the woman in the decision-making process.

Women with a family history of breast cancer should be referred to regional genetic services. *Primary care has an important role in identifying and referring at-risk patients.*[31]

It is becoming apparent that oral and transdermal administration routes for oestrogens in HRT for menopausal women have different risk-benefit profiles.[32] The risk of venous thromboembolism (VTE) is higher with an oral rather than transdermal route. The nested case control study using the UK General Practice Research Database confirmed that oral users of HRT had a higher rate of stroke than non-users.[32] Use of transdermal HRT containing a low dose of oestrogen did not increase the risk of stroke.

It is a well-known fact that menopause is associated with a rise in cardiovascular disease. The authors concluded that a more rapid menopausal transition was associated with a higher rate of preclinical cardiovascular disease progression.[33]

Local oestrogen is highly effective for the management of vulvo-vaginal atrophy and sexual dysfunction and can be used long term.

Initial assessment

- Take a history and assess menopausal status.
- Check for contraindications to HRT therapy.
- Check weight and BMI.
- Check blood pressure.
- Give lifestyle advice.
- Check that regular cervical screening is taking place.
- Advise the woman about breast awareness. Check that mammography screening is in place if over 50 years. Mammography is not needed before commencing HRT unless the woman is at high risk of breast cancer.[34]

Benefits of HRT

- Improvement in vasomotor symptoms within a few weeks of commencing therapy.
- Improvement of vaginal symptoms occurs within 3 months.
- Osteoporosis prevention: the bone protection lasts as long as HRT is taken. Evidence that HRT prevents fracture is less strong. Observational studies show a reduction in fracture risk of 65%.[35]
- Unproven benefits: primary prevention of CVD.
- Dementia and cognitive function: the evidence is conflicting and HRT should not be used for this purpose.

Risks of HRT

- Endometrial cancer.
- Venous thromboembolism.

- Breast cancer.
- Coronary heart disease and stroke if initiated in older women.

Contraindications

Absolute contraindications:
- acute-phase myocardial infarction
- pulmonary embolism or DVT
- pregnancy
- active breast cancer
- active endometrial cancer
- undiagnosed breast lump
- un-investigated vaginal bleeding
- severe active liver disease.

Relative contraindications:
- diabetes
- gall bladder disease
- fibroids: HRT may cause enlargement of fibroids
- endometriosis: refer to gynaecologist
- past history of breast or endometrial cancer: refer to gynaecologist
- family history of thromboembolic disease: offer thrombophilia screening before commencing therapy.

How to address the side effects of HRT

Oestrogenic side effects such as nausea, headaches and breast tenderness:
- trial of a lower dose
- switch to transdermal patch from oral therapy
- persevere as this may settle with time (3 months)
- use oestradiol rather than conjugate equine oestrogens (CEE).

Progestogenic side effects such as acne, bloated feeling and pre menstrual like symptoms:
- try a different progestogen
- decrease the duration of progestogen to 7 or 10 days
- use Mirena coil instead.

Breakthrough bleeding on continuous combined HRT:
- explain to patients that the risk of bleeding is 40% in the first 4–6 months
- change to transdermal HRT
- try a more androgenic progestogen containing HRT
- combine with Mirena coil.

Follow up of women on HRT:
- See after 3 months, then 6-monthly.
- Check for compliance, bleeding pattern and side effects.
- Check weight, BMI and blood pressure.
- Enquire about smoking and alcohol intake.
- Check patient is up to date with smears and mammograms.

Risk of breast cancer
- Use of combined HRT is associated with an increased risk of breast cancer that increases with duration of use. In post menopausal women the estimated absolute risk of breast cancer is 30 cases per 10 000 women per year in non users as compared to 38 cases per 10 000 women per year (averaged over 5 years).[36]
- Long-term use (more than 5 years) is associated with a small increase in cases of breast cancer.[37]
- Once a woman has stopped HRT for 5 years or more she loses excess risk.[36]

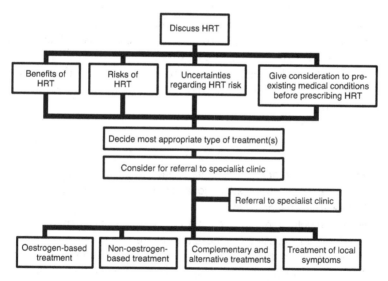

FIGURE 20.1 HRT algorithm
Source: Map of Medicine Menopause pathway. www.gponline.com/Clinical/article/1026538/hrt-use-menopausal-women/

Management of premature menopause
HRT is the mainstay of treatment until the age of natural menopause; that is 52 years as recommended by the BMS.[38] HRT should be tailored to the needs of the individual. Treatment for women with an intact uterus commonly

involves sequential HRT or the combined contraceptive pill. The type of oestrogen – whether 17b-estradiol or ethinyl estradiol – has no effect on the endometrium or the lipid profile.[39]

Women who have had a hysterectomy will only need oestrogen replacement therapy. Lack of libido can be improved with concomitant testosterone.

Women with menopause after treatment for cancer face fertility problems. They need to be referred to a specialist fertility centre for cryopreservation of oocytes or embryos.[40] Patients with Turner's syndrome can also achieve similar pregnancy rates as those with oocyte donations. But they have a higher rate of miscarriage, hypertension and pre-eclampsia.[1]

Quality of life (QOL) at menopause

Following the first publication of the Women's Health Initiative (WHI) study in 2002,[41] it was suggested that menopause having no impact on mortality is not a significant concern. This resulted in the cessation of the Women's International Study of Long Duration of Oestrogens after the Menopause (WISDOM) trial in October 2002. This had intended to be a 10-year trial. WISDOM evaluated (QOL) using general and menopause-specific assessment tools. The WISDOM paper tells us that HRT relieves symptoms and improves QOL. This benefit is greatest for those most affected.[42] WHI findings in respect of coronary heart disease have been adjudicated and reanalysed.[43] Prescribers are now able to advise women that there is no increase in cardiac risk if HRT is started close to menopause, when a woman is most symptomatic.

KEY POINTS

- Menopause is complicated and its impact on an individual depends on genetic, ethnic, cultural, educational, economic, environmental, family, lifestyle and situational factors.
- HRT is the gold standard treatment for menopausal vasomotor symptoms, especially when these are severe.
- Women using combined HRT for >5 years have a slightly increased risk of breast cancer, but this is not seen with shorter duration of use.
- Women who do not wish to take HRT should be given lifestyle advice to help alleviate their vasomotor symptoms.
- Phytooestrogens such as red clover isoflavones have some evidence to support their use for vasomotor and mood symptoms.
- Exercise is a safe and effective way of preventing bone loss in postmenopausal women.
- Half of postmenopausal women will suffer a fracture during their

lifetime, mainly due to osteoporosis, but many do not receive appropriate assessment and treatment.

- The clinical needs of patients with premature menopause are both physical and psychological and must be managed appropriately.
- Cultural perceptions of the menopause as a positive or a negative experience vary greatly. Non-white women consistently report fewer symptoms.
- An age-appropriate dose of HRT – higher for younger women and lower for older women – is crucial to maximise efficacy and minimise risks.
- Global risks of HRT cannot be generically applied because there are differences between the routes of administration and dose.
- Transdermal HRT should be considered in older age groups or women with risk factors for VTE or stroke.

Patient information

Cancer research UK www.cancerhelp.org.uk

Macmillan Cancer Support www.macmillan.org.uk

Daisy Network Premature Menopause Support Group. Can provide psychological support

www.daisynetwork.org.uk

National Osteoporosis Society. www.nos.org.uk

Guidance for elderly patients with hip fractures www.nhfd.co.uk

Patient information from Women's Health Concern www.womens-health-concern.org

Useful websites

For GPs

Department of Health. Fracture prevention services: an economic evaluation; November 2009: www.dh.gov.uk/en/Publicationsandstatistics/Publications/PublicationsPolicyAndGuidance/DH_110098

FRAX: www.shef.ac.uk/FRAX

International Menopause Society consensus statement: updated recommendations on postmenopausal hormone therapy; 2007: www.imsociety.org/ims_recommendations.php

Million Women Study www.millionwomenstudy.org

National Osteoporosis Guideline Group: www.shef.ac.uk/NOGG

New map of medicine menopause pathway: www.mapofmedicine.com

NICE. Osteoporosis: primary prevention (TA160): http://guidance.nice.org.uk/TA160

NICE. Osteoporosis: secondary prevention including strontium ranelate (TA161): http://guidance.nice.org.uk/TA161

NICE. Osteoporotic fractures: denosumab (TA204): http://guidance.nice.org.uk/TA204

Women's health initiative: www.nhlbi.nih.gov/whi/

References

1 Rees M, Purdie DW. *Management of the menopause: the handbook of the British Menopause Society.* London: RSM Press; 2006.

2 Pitkin J, Rees MC, Gray S, *et al.* Management of premature menopause. *Menopause Int.* 2007; **13**(1): 44–5.

3 Ossewaarde ME, Bots ML, Verbeek AL, *et al.* Age at menopause, cause-specific mortality and total life expectancy. *Epidemiology.* 2005; **16**(4): 556–62.

4 Gold EB, Block G, Crawford S, *et al.* Lifestyle and demographic factors in relation to vasomotor symptoms: baseline results from the Study of Women's Health Across the Nations. *Am J Epidemiol.* 2004; **159**(12): 1189–99. www.ncbi.nlm.gov >Journal List >NIHPA Author Manuscript

5 Thurston RC. *Menopausal Medicine.* 2009; **17**(1): s1–s6.

6 Avis NE, Kaufert PA, Lock M, *et al.* The evolution of menopausal symptoms. In: Burger HG, editor. *The Menopause.* London: Elsevier; 1993.

7 Archer DF, Dupont CM, Constantine GD, *et al.* Desvenlafaxine for the treatment of vasomotor symptoms associated with menopause: a double-blind, randomized, placebo-controlled trial of efficacy and safety. *Am J Obstet Gynecol.* 2009; **200**(3): 238e1–e10.

8 Rufford BD, Jacobs IJ. Royal College of Obstetricians and Gynaecologists. Ovarian cysts in postmenopausal women. Green-top guideline 34. London: RCOG; 2003.

9 Valentin L, Skoog L, Epstein E. Frequency and type of adnexal lesions in autopsy material from postmenopausal women: ultrasound study with histological correlation. *Ultrasound Obstet Gynecol.* 2003; **22**(3): 284–9.

10 Cohen I, Potlog-Nahari C, Shapira J, *et al.* Simple ovarian cysts in postmenopausal patients with breast carcinoma treated with tamoxifen: long-term follow-up. *Radiology.* 2003; **227**(3): 844–8.

11 Canonico M, Oger E, Conrad J, *et al.* Obesity and risk of venous thromboembolism among postmenopausal women: differential impact of hormone therapy by route of estrogen administration. *J Thromb Haemost.* 2006; **4**(6); 1259–65.

12 The Information Centre. Statistics on obesity, physical activity and diet. NHS; 2008. Available at: www.ic.nhs.uk/pubs/opadjan08 (accessed 16 December 2012).

13 Vaidya D, Becker DM, Bittner V. Aging, menopause and ischaemic heart disease mortality in England, Wales and the United States: modelling study of national mortality data. *BMJ.* 2011; 343: d5170.

14 Jebb SA, Ahern AL, Olson AD, *et al.* Best approach to weight loss: primary care physician referring to Weight Watchers. *Lancet.* 2011; 378: 1485–92. Available at: www.weightwatchers.co.uk/util/art/index_art.aspx?tabnum=1&art_id=54351&sc=3046

15 National Institute for Health and Clinical Excellence. Hypertension: Management of Hypertension in Adults in Primary Care. NICE guideline 34. London: NIHCE; 2006. www.nice.org.uk/guidance/CG34

16 National Institute for Health and Clinical Excellence. Lipid Modification: NICE guideline 67. London: NIHCE; 2008. www.nice.org.uk/guidance/CG67.

17 Management of type 2 diabetes: summary of updated NICE guidance. *BMJ*. **336**(7656): 1306–8.

18 National Institute for Health and Clinical Excellence. Type 2 Diabetes: Newer Agents (practical update of CG 66). NICE guideline 87. London: NIHCE; 2009. www.nice.org.uk/guidance/CG87

19 Howe TE, Shea B, Dawson LJ, *et al*. Exercise for preventing and treating osteoporosis in post menopausal women. Cochrane Database Syst Rev. 2011; 7: CD000333.

20 Nutraingredients.com. Women opt for natural menopause treatment. Available online at: www.nutraingredients.com/Research/Women-opt-for-natural-menopause-treatment

21 Nedrow A, Miller J, Walker M, *et al*. Complementary and alternative therapies for the management of menopause related symptoms. *Arch Intern Med*. 2006; **166**(14): 1453–65.

22 MHRA. Black cohosh: UK Public Assessment Report. Available at: www.mhra.gov.uk/home/groups/es-herbal/documents/websiteresources/con2024279.pdf (accessed 25 February 2013).

23 Grube B, Walper A, Wheatley D. St John's wort extract: efficacy for menopausal symptoms of psychological origin. *Adv Ther*. 1999; **16**(4): 177–86.

24 Uebelhack R, Bloher JW, Graubaum HJ, *et al*. Black cohosh and St John's wort for climacteric complaints. *Obstet Gynecol*. 2006; **107**(2 Pt 1): 247–55.

25 Stevenson JC. Coronary heart disease and menopause management: the swinging pendulum of HRT. *Atherosclerosis*. 2009; **207**(2): 336–40.

26 Lindh-Astrand L, Bixo M, Hirschberg AL, *et al*. A randomised controlled study of taper-down or abrupt discontinuation of hormone therapy in women treated for vasomotor symptoms. *Menopause*. 2010; **17**(1): 72–9.

27 Committee on Safety of Medicines. Further advice on safety of HRT: risk: benefit unfavourable for first-line use in prevention of osteoporosis. CEM/CMO/2003/19. Available at: www.mhra.gov.uk/home/groups/pl-p/documents/websiteresources/con019496.pdf (accessed 16 December 2012).

28 The Women's Health Initiative steering committee. Effects of conjugated equine oestrogen in postmenopausal women with hysterectomy: the Women's Health Initiative randomised controlled trial. *JAMA*. 2004; 291: 1701–12.

29 Beral V. Million Women Study Collaborators. Breast cancer and hormone replacement therapy in the Million Women Study. *Lancet*. 2003; 362: 419–27.

30 Kokcu A, Cetinkaya MB, Yanik F, *et al*. The comparison of effects of tibolone and conjugated estrogen-medroxyprogesterone acetate therapy on sexual performance in postmenopausal women. *Maturitas*. 2000; **36**(1): 75–80.

31 National Institute for Health and Clinical Excellence. Familial breast cancer: NICE guideline 41. London: NIHCE; 2006. http://guidance.nice.org.uk/CG41

32 Renoux C, Dellaniello S, Garbe E, *et al*. Transdermal and oral hormone replacement therapy and the risk of stroke: a nested case-control study. *BMJ*. 2010; 340: c2519.

33 Johnson BD, Dwyer KM, Stanczyk FZ, *et al*. The relationship of menopausal status

and rapid menopausal transition with carotid intima-media thickness progression in women. *J Clin Endocrinol Metab.* 2010; **95**(9): 4432–40.

34 Hope S, Rees M and Brockie J. *Hormone Replacement Therapy: a guide for primary care.* Oxford: Oxford University Press; 1999.

35 Royal College of Physicians and the Bone and Tooth Society of Great Britain. Osteoporosis: clinical guidelines for prevention and treatment. RCP London. www.rcplondon.ac.uk

36 New Zealand Guidelines Group. Best practice evidence-based guidelines for the appropriate prescribing of hormone replacement therapy. New Zealand Guidelines Group; 2001. www.medsafe.govt.nz/downloads/hrt_summary_web. pdf

37 Collaborative Group on Hormonal Factors in Breast Cancer. Breast cancer and hormone replacement therapy: collaborative reanalysis of data from 51 epidemiological studies of 52,705 women with breast cancer and 108,411 women without breast cancer. *Lancet.* 1997; **350**(9084): 1047–59.

38 Committee on Safety of Medicines. Further advice on safety of HRT: risk: benefit unfavourable for first-line use in prevention of osteoporosis. CEM/CMO/2003/19. Available at: www.mhra.gov.uk/home/groups/pl-p/documents/websiteresources/con019496.pdf (accessed 15 December 2012).

39 Guttmann H, Weiner Z, Nikolski E, *et al.* Choosing an oestrogen replacement therapy in young adult women with Turner syndrome. *Clin Endocrinol (Oxf).* 2001; **54**(2): 159–64.

40 Beerendonk CC, Braat DD. Present and future options for the preservation of fertility in female adolescents with cancer. *Endocr Dev.* 2005; 8: 166–75.

41 Writing Group for the Women's Health Initiative Investigators. Risks and benefits of oestrogen plus progestin in healthy postmenopausal women: principal results from the Women's Health Initiative randomised controlled trial. *JAMA.* 2002; **288**(3): 321–33.

42 Welton AJ, Vickers MR, Kim J, *et al.* Health related quality of life after combined hormone replacement therapy: randomised controlled trial. *BMJ.* 2008; 337: a1190.

43 Rossouw JE, Prentice RL, Manson JE, *et al.* Postmenopausal hormone therapy and risk of cardiovascular disease by age and years since menopause. *JAMA.* 2007; 297: 1465–77.

21

Understanding gynaecological ultrasound scan

Ultrasound has become a part of routine clinical practice. However, it must be remembered that it should only complement rather than replace clinical practice. A thorough medical history and clinical examination such as abdominal palpation and vaginal examination where appropriate, will ensure appropriate interpretation of the gynaecological ultrasound scan (USS). It should not be the only modality whereby referral to secondary care is made.

In gynaecological ultrasounds, a transvaginal ultrasound will provide optimum images in most cases, as the ultrasound probe is close to the uterus and adnexae and therefore provides better images. Contrary to common belief, a vaginal ultrasound is not as uncomfortable as an abdominal ultrasound as, for the latter, a full bladder is required, which is uncomfortable in itself and is accentuated by pressure on the abdomen by the probe. In obese patients, a transvaginal option is the preferred modality.

Uterus

Normal anatomy

The uterus is anteverted (tilted forwards) in the majority of instances. In a small percentage the uterus may be retroverted (tilted backwards). This is not associated with any pathology. The description of the size of the uterus should correlate with the clinical examination. One often comes across reports mentioning a 'bulky uterus'. This is not of much clinical significance and may be associated with parity, small fibroids or adenomyosis. The patient's history and findings on abdominal and vaginal examination are more relevant than emphasis on this particular aspect in the report.

The endometrium changes according to the stage in the menstrual cycle.

At the beginning of the menstrual cycle, the endometrium is at its thinnest. During the follicular phase, the endometrium becomes thicker and manifests as a 'triple echo' just prior to ovulation[1] (*see* Figure 21.1).

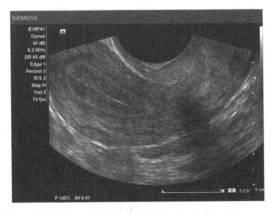

FIGURE 21.1 Triple echo pattern of the endometrium in the pre-ovulatory follicular phase

During the post-ovulatory phase, the endometrium becomes hyperechoeic, indicative of a secretory endometrium (*see* Figure 21.2).

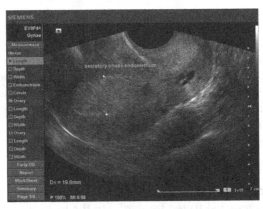

FIGURE 21.2 Hyperechoeic secretory phase endometrium

Due to the changes of the endometrium during the menstrual cycle in a woman's reproductive life, an ultrasound report describing endometrial thickness in the reproductive age group is not of much clinical value when compared to the postmenopausal phase.

During the postmenopausal phase, the endometrium has a uniform ultrasound morphology because there are no cyclical hormonal changes. It

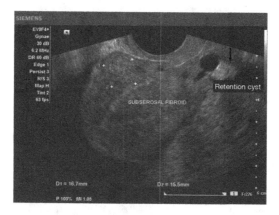

FIGURE 21.3 Retention cyst (Nabothian follicle cervix)

is thin and hyperechoeic, measuring no more than 4–5 mm thick.[2,3] In some instances there may be a small amount of fluid in the cavity, which may be a normal finding indicative of a collection of secretions in the uterine cavity associated with a stenotic cervix seen in the postmenopausal phase.

With regard to the cervix, it is not uncommon to note retention cysts (Nabothian follicles) on an ultrasound scan. No action is required in such reports (*see* Figure 21.3).

Uterine abnormalities on ultrasound scan
Congenital uterine abnormalities
Anomalies are often encountered as an incidental finding in women who attend for pelvic scan and it is often unclear how these anomalies are managed in asymptomatic women. In women in the reproductive age group who present with recurrent miscarriage, it is suggested that there may be an association with uterine abnormalities, although clear evidence regarding the benefits of treatment is lacking.[4] In such cases, it may be worth seeking the opinion of a gynaecologist. These anomalies may vary from a subseptate uterus to a bicornuate uterus. These anomalies can be enhanced by the 3D ultrasound scan (*see* Figures 21.4 and 21.5).

Uterine fibroids
Uterine fibroids are the most common uterine abnormality presenting in the reproductive age group. They could be an incidental ultrasound finding in women who attend for a pelvic scan. It is the presenting complaint such as menorrhagia, dysmenorrhoea or pressure symptoms on surrounding organs such as urinary frequency, as well as the location of the fibroid (*see* Figure 21.6) rather than its presence, which will determine referral to

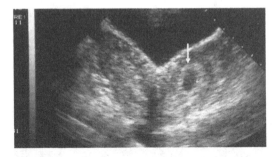

FIGURE 21.4 Bicornuate uterus with GS in one horn (2D)

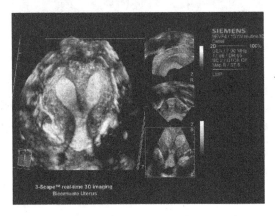

FIGURE 21.5 Bicornuate uterus (3D)

secondary care. Intramural fibroids rarely cause problems unless they are large (usually greater than 5 cm) and associated with symptoms as described above. Subserous fibroids also rarely cause symptoms unless they are significantly large, causing pressure-related symptoms (*see* Figure 21.8). The most significant of all the fibroids are the submucous fibroids which cause menorrhagia. Type 0 fibroids, where the majority of the fibroid is in the uterine cavity, are most suitable for hysteroscopic resection as a day-case procedure (*see* Figure 21.7).[5] Some type 1 fibroids (50% in the uterine cavity and 50% intramural) may also be suitable for endometrial resection.

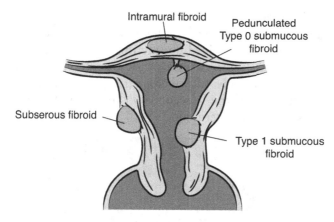

FIGURE 21.6 Location of uterine fibroids

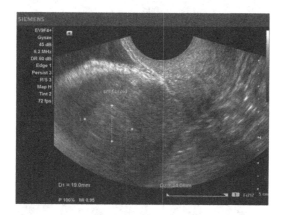

FIGURE 21.7 Intracavitory submucous fibroid

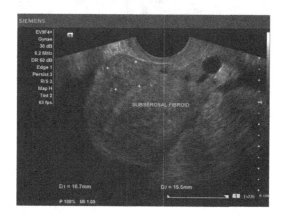

FIGURE 21.8 Subserous fibroid

Endometrial polyps

These are discrete focal thickenings of the endometrium and may be associated with intermenstrual bleeding, menorrhagia or postmenopausal bleeding. A characteristic feeder vessel or pedicle artery sign on application of colour Doppler is indicative of an endometrial polyp (*see* Figures 12.9 and 21.10).[6] In such cases referral to secondary care should be considered for removal or resection via hysteroscopy.

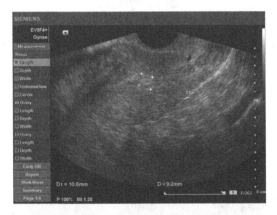

FIGURE 21.9 Endometrial polyp in uterine cavity

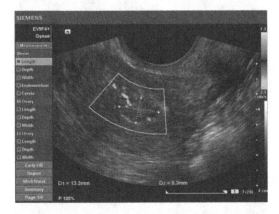

FIGURE 21.10 Doppler showing the typical feeder vessel to the uterine polyp

Ovaries

Normal anatomy

Ovarian morphology changes during the menstrual cycle. During folliculo-genesis, of the 3–11 follicles in the ovary (*see* Figure 21.11), one follicle known as the dominant follicle can grow up to 18–22 mm in size.[7] (*see* Figure 21.12). Hence for a woman in the reproductive age group, descriptions of 'cysts' should correlate with the stage in the menstrual cycle. In the luteal phase, following ovulation the follicle ruptures to become the corpus luteum, which may have a typical perivascular ring on Doppler (*see* Figure 21.13). Bleeding into the corpus luteum may explain the presence of echoes on USS. These are physiological changes that are commonly reported on ultrasound scans.

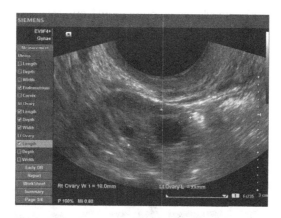

FIGURE 21.11 Normal right ovary with a few follicles

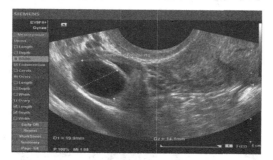

FIGURE 21.12 Dominant follicle on day 13 in the menstrual cycle

Functional physiological cysts (*see* Figure 21.14) are usually less than 5 cm in diameter with thin smooth walls and echolucent echoes typical of clear fluid-filled cysts.[8] An example of a functional ovarian cyst that may be mistaken for an endometrioma is a haemorrhagic corpus luteum (*see* Figure 21.15).

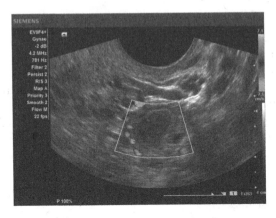

FIGURE 21.13 Typical postovulatory corpus luteum Doppler showing a perivascular ring

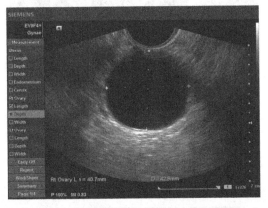

FIGURE 21.14 A simple ovarian cyst

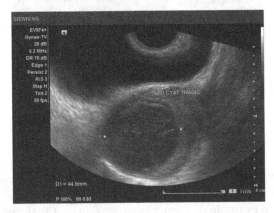

FIGURE 21.15 Spider web appearance of a typical haemorrhagic cyst

It typically contains web-like material (fibrin and blood clot) which tends to regress in 2–3 months. A rescan in 3 months may show disappearance of the cyst. Women known to have ovarian cysts present with acute pain, and the diagnosis of a torsion, rupture or haemorrhage should be considered.

There is no need to do a serum CA-125 test in premenopausal women when an ultrasound diagnosis of a simple ovarian cyst is made. If women present with a complex ovarian mass under the age of 40, the possibility of germ cell tumours should be considered and tumour markers such as LDH (lactic dehydrogenase), alphafetoprotein and human chorionic gonadotrophin should be performed. CA-125 is not very reliable in differentiating benign from malignant ovarian masses in premenopausal women because of the increased false positive rates.[9]

CA-125 may be raised in endometriosis, fibroids, adenomyosis and pelvic infection. In the above conditions, the CA-125 is marginally raised (less than 200 units/ml) while in malignancy the levels are significantly raised.

In women who present during the postmenopausal stage with ovarian cysts, a CA-125 and referral to secondary care should be made. In such cases the RMI 1 (Risk of Malignancy Index) is applied and the patient categorised as low/intermediate or high risk.[10]

RMI 1 combines 3 pre-surgical features: Ultrasound score (1 for each finding) × menopausal status (1 for premenopausal and 3 for post menopausal) × CA125 (measured in IU/ml).

Low risk = 25

Medium risk = 25–250

High risk = >250

Conservative management may be advocated in the postmenopausal patient who, following referral to secondary care for a simple cyst with low risk, has had three scans 4 months apart – if the cyst has not increased in size, then she can be discharged on the advice of the secondary care clinician.

Transvaginal ultrasound scans are useful in women presenting with adnexal masses on clinical examination.

Dermoid cysts

Characteristic features include a mixture of intensely echogenic areas from hair and sebum to prominent echogenic dots in cyst fluid (*see* Figure 21.16).

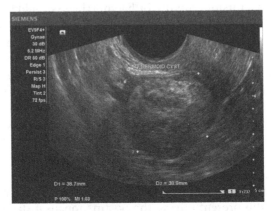

FIGURE 21.16 Dermoid cyst showing hyperechoeic areas

Endometriomas

Endometriomas characteristically show a typical 'ground glass' appearance on ultrasound (*see* Figure 21.17). One or more solid foci may be present in the endometrioma, which may represent blood clot or fibrin. The differential diagnosis includes dermoid cysts, adenofibroma and haemorrhagic cysts. These patients should be referred to secondary care. Further management depends on the patient's history.

Patients with pelvic pain may need removal of the endometrioma either laparoscopically or via a laparotomy. Tumour markers such as CA-125 may be raised in this condition.

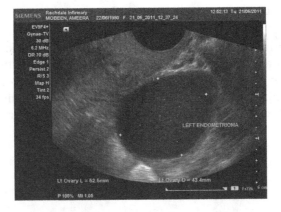

FIGURE 21.17 Endometrioma ovary

Incidental findings of ovarian cysts on USS

Many ovarian cysts that may have previously been undetected may be picked up on USS if these scans are carried out on asymptomatic women. A conservative approach should be considered in small cysts (usually less than 5 cm) with benign features in asymptomatic women, as surgery is associated with risks. An important point to remember is that USS should be requested only if clinically indicated. USS should not be used as a substitute for a good clinical history and examination. Cysts larger than 25 mm are found in 7% of premenopausal asymptomatic women and cysts larger than 15 mm are found in 7% of asymptomatic postmenopausal women. Hence, even if cysts are detected on USS in patients with a history of pelvic pain, this finding may not be necessarily related to the patient's symptoms and other causes such as irritable bowel syndrome, urinary tract infections, etc. should be excluded.[11]

Polycystic ovaries

Polycystic ovaries should manifest at least one of the following features:
- 12 or more follicles measuring 2–9 mm in diameter
- increased ovarian volume (greater than 10 cm³).

A diagnosis of polycystic ovarian syndrome should be made only if two of the following three criteria are met:
- hyperandrogenism
- chronic anovulation
- polycystic ovaries on USS.[12]

The isolated finding of polycystic ovaries on its own does not constitute a syndrome, and referral to secondary care should be based on clinical history such as oligomenorrhoea or subfertility due to anovulation (*see* Figure 21.18).

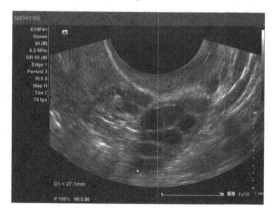

FIGURE 21.18 Polycystic ovary

TABLE 21.1 USS features between SIMPLE and COMPLEX ovarian cysts

SIMPLE CYSTS	COMPLEX CYSTS
Size less than 5 cm	Size more than 5 cm
Unilocular	Multilocular
Thin septae	Thick septae
Absence of papillary projections	Presence of papillary projections

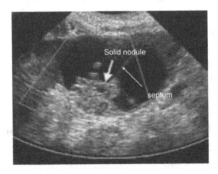

FIGURE 21.19 Complex ovarian cyst

Fallopian tubes

The fallopian tubes are not normally seen on USS, but may be identified in conditions such as tubo-ovarian masses, or hydrosalpinges. The typical appearance in hydrosalpinges are 'sausage-shaped' lesions (*see* Figure 21.20) or incomplete septae (cog wheel appearance) (*see* Figure 21.21).

These lesions may be picked up in patients presenting with pelvic pain, in which case referral to secondary care should be considered. In women undergoing treatment for in vitro fertilisation, the presence of hydrosalpinges may be embryotoxic and referral to secondary care for salpingectomy should be considered.

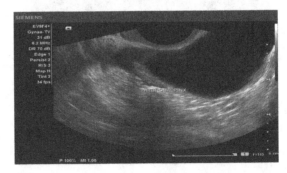

FIGURE 21.20 Hydrosalpinx

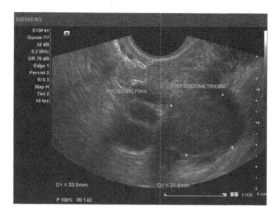

FIGURE 21.21 Cogwheel appearance of a hydrosalpinx

Fluid in the Pouch of Douglas (POD)

This is a common finding on ultrasound in women in the late follicular phase of the menstrual cycle and early luteal phase. At this stage the amount of fluid may be around 15–25 ml (*see* Figure 21.22). It is not possible to give an exact cut-off point for what is normal, but fluid outside the POD is unusual (fluid between the uterus and bladder is abnormal) (*see* Figure 21.23). It should be noted that fluid in the POD in postmenopausal women is unusual.[13]

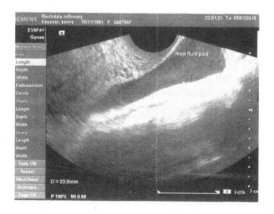

FIGURE 21.22 Fluid in the Pouch of Douglas (POD)

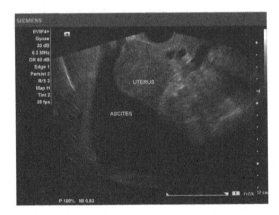

FIGURE 21.23 Fluid in front of the uterus (behind the bladder) in a woman who presented to A&E with metastatic ovarian cancer and ascites on scan was noted

KEY POINTS

- Ultrasound findings should be interpreted in conjunction with the patient's history and clinical examination.
- Uterine enlargement is nearly always due to fibroids, and the sonographer will give the measurements and describe the position. Fibroids do not usually need a referral unless they are causing symptoms.
- The appearance and thickness of the endometrium varies with different stages of the menstrual cycle.
- In postmenopausal women presenting with vaginal bleeding, an endometrial thickness of less than 4 mm on ultrasound is unlikely to reveal any endometrial pathology.
- In asymptomatic premenopausal women presenting with simple ovarian cysts on ultrasound, a size of less than 5 cm does not normally require referral to secondary care.
- It is reassuring to note that if ovaries are not seen on ultrasound scan, it is unlikely to reveal any pathology.
- Tubes are usually not seen – if visible there is usually a pathology such as hydrosalpinx.

References

1 Ritchie WG. Sonographic evaluation of normal and induced ovulation. *Radiology.* 1986; 161: 1–10.

2 Merz E, Miric-Tesanic D, Bahlman F, *et al.* Sonographic size of uterus and ovaries in pre and postmenopausal women. *Ultrasound Obstetric Gynecol.* 1996; 7: 38–42.

3 Sladkevicius P, Valentin L, Marsal K. Transvaginal grey scale and Doppler ultrasound examinations of the uterus and ovaries in healthy postmenopausal women. *Ultrasound Obstet Gynecol.* 1995; 6: 81–90.

4 Salim R, Regan L, Woelfer B, *et al.* A comparative study of the morphology of congenital uterine anomalies in women with or without a history of recurrent first trimester miscarriage. *Hum Reprod.* 2003; 1: 162–6.

5 Vercellini P, Cortesi I, Oldham S, *et al.* The role of transvaginal ultrasonography and outpatient hysteroscopy in the evaluation of the patient with menorrhagia. *Hum Reprod.* 1997; 12: 1768–71.

6 Timmer D, Deprest J, Bourne T, *et al.* A randomised trial on the use of ultrasound or office hysteroscopy for endometrial assessment in postmenopausal women with breast cancer who are treated with tamoxifen. *Am J Obstet Gynecol.* 1998; 179: 62–70.

7 Bakos O, Lundkvist O, Wide L, *et al.* Ultrasonographic and hormonal description of the normal ovulatory cycle. *Acta Obstet Gynecol Scand.* 1994; 73: 790–6.

8 Timmerman D, Valentin L, Bourne TH, *et al.* Terms, definitions and measurements to describe the sonographic features of adnexal tumours: a consensus opinion from the International Ovarian Tumour Analysis (IOTA) group. *Ultrasound Obstet Gynecol.* 2000; 16: 500–5.

9 Royal College of Obstetricians and Gynaecologists (RGOG). Management of suspected ovarian masses in premenopausal women. Green-top guideline 62. RCOG; 2011.

10 Royal College of Obstetricians and Gynaecologists (RGOG). Management of ovarian cysts in postmenopausal women. Green-top guideline 34. RCOG; 2003.

11 Valentin L, Akram D. The natural history of adnexal cysts incidentally detected at transvaginal ultrasound in postmenopausal women. *Ultrasound Obstet Gynecol.* 2002; 20: 174–80.

12 Rotterdam ESHRE/ARSM-Sponsored PCOS Consensus Workshop Group. Revised 2003 consensus on diagnostic criteria and long-term health risks related to polycystic ovary syndrome. *Hum Reprod.* 2004; 19: 41–7.

13 Merz E, Miric-Tesanic D, Bahlman F, *et al.* Sonographic size of uterus and ovaries in pre and postmenopausal women. *Ultrasound Obstet Gynecol.* 1996; 7: 38–42.

22

Polycystic ovary syndrome

Polycystic ovary syndrome (PCOS), formerly known as Stein–Leventhal syndrome, is one of the commonest endocrine disorders, affecting women during their reproductive years.

DEFINITION

PCOS is defined as detection of polycystic ovaries by ultrasound scan. Polycystic ovaries are larger ovaries and have twice the number of follicles (small cysts). The disorder is characterised by anovulation and hyperandrogenism with clinical symptoms of anovulation, irregular cycles, acne, infertility, hirsutism and obesity.

A consensus definition using precise diagnostic criteria should be used when diagnosing PCOS to facilitate effective patient care and robust clinical research.[21] The 1990 National Institutes of Health (NIH) preliminary consensus definition has now been replaced by a Rotterdam European Society for Human Reproduction and Embryology (ESHRE) and American Society of Reproductive Medicine (ASRM) PCOS Consensus Workshop Group definition.[1]

This suggests a broader definition for PCOS with two of the three following criteria being diagnostic of the condition:

- polycystic ovaries (either 12 or more peripheral follicles or increased ovarian volume (greater than 10 cm^3)
- oligo- and/or anovulation resulting in irregular menstruation, amenorrhoea and ovulation related infertility
- clinical and or biochemical signs of hyperandrogensim.

The new diagnostic criteria have affected the value of a number of systematic reviews, as the majority were based on the 1990 NIH criteria (oligo- or anovulation and biochemical or clinical signs of hyperandrogenism such as

---

hirsutism, acne or male-pattern hair loss). The recent broadened Rotterdam criteria have incorporated the morphologic appearance of ovaries[2] as one of the possible traits of the syndrome.

Prevalence

Polycystic ovaries occur in 20%–25% of women during their reproductive years. The prevalence is thought to be higher in south-Asian women. Women from south Asia have worse symptoms, worse hormonal and metabolic disturbances and a greater chance of developing type 2 diabetes.

Hormonal changes

One third of women have no hormonal abnormality. The hormonal changes in PCOS are:
- raised concentration of luteinising hormone (LH)
- raised concentration of testosterone.

Primary care management

History

Having polycystic ovaries does not mean polycystic ovary syndrome is present. Six to seven per cent of women with polycystic ovaries have PCOS. The commonest cause of irregular menstruation is polycystic ovaries.[3] A woman with PCOS presents with:
- irregular periods or no periods at all
- difficulty becoming pregnant
- hirsutism (hair in the midline involving lip and chin is characteristic of hirsutism, as is male-pattern hair loss on the scalp, hair in the lateral margins of the lip, hair on the sternum and pubic hair rising up to the umbilicus; hirsutism is characterised by coarse terminal hair rather than fine vellus hair)
- overweight: BMI >30; 40% of women with confirmed PCOS are overweight
- oily skin and acne
- mood swings/depression.

Diagnosis

- Truncal obesity BMI greater than 30.
- Elevated level of LH >12 iu/L or three times FSH level when carried out during menstruation. FSH concentration is normal. If the patient has amenorrhoea, then FSH and LH can be measured at any time.

- Prolactin level: this may be mildly elevated in PCOS but high levels (more than 1000 mu/L) should raise suspicion of a pituitary tumour.
- Raised fasting blood glucose or impaired glucose tolerance especially in obese women.
- Raised triglyceride level.
- Serum testosterone: mild elevation suggests PCOS. If the value is more than twice the normal value, this raises suspicion of an androgenic metabolic disorder or a tumour.
- Sex hormone binding globulin: this protein binds testosterone and a low level of SHBG results in increased concentrations of free testosterone.
- The ultrasound scan (USS): the USS is the main diagnostic aid to study the morphology of the ovaries.

The criteria for ultrasound diagnosis of PCOS has recently been revised in light of improved ultrasound technology and better understanding of the condition.[4]

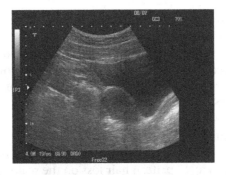

FIGURE 22.1 Transabdominal scan

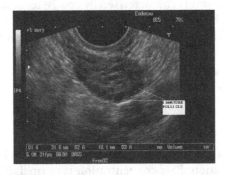

FIGURE 22.2 Transvaginal scan findings: right ovary

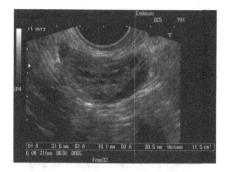

FIGURE 22.3 Transvaginal scan findings: right ovary

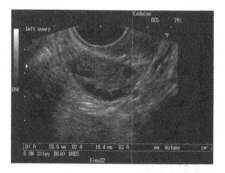

FIGURE 22.4 Transvaginal scan findings: left ovary

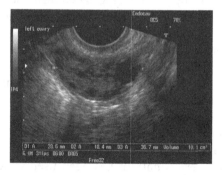

FIGURE 22.5 Transvaginal scan findings: left ovary

The diagnosis can be supported when one or more of the following features are demonstrated:

- 12 or more follicles (3–12 mm diameter) are present in an ovary[5] either peripherally or diffusely arranged)
- ovarian volume is over 10 cm³ (when no follicles measuring over 10 mm in diameter are present).

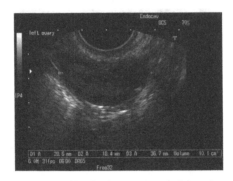

FIGURE 22.6 Transvaginal scan: uterus. Endometrium, day 6

Only a single ovary need be affected to make the diagnosis. If a large follicle is present (over 10 mm) then the volume should be calculated on a repeat scan when the ovary is quiescent to prevent overestimation of ovarian volume.

Bright ovarian stroma relative to the myometrium is no longer an essential part of the diagnosis but is specific to the condition and provides supporting evidence in the presence of essential features.

History of diagnosis of PCOS

Historically, detection of the polycystic ovary required visualisation of the ovaries at laparotomy and histological confirmation following biopsy. Further studies identified the association of certain endocrine abnormalities in women with the histological evidence of polycystic ovaries. Biochemical criteria became the mainstay for diagnosis. Raised serum levels of LH, testosterone and androstenedione, in association with low or normal levels of FSH, were described as an endocrine profile which many believed to be diagnostic of polycystic ovary syndrome.

Presentation of the syndrome is varied as there is considerable hetero-geneity of symptoms and signs amongst women with PCOS. Many studies have shown that most present an ultrasound picture of polycystic ovaries.[5]

Ultrasonographic examination[6] has been used widely for evaluating PCOS. Two types of PCOS have been identified: peripheral cystic pattern (PCP) and general cystic pattern (GCP). In PCP, small cysts are aligned in the subcapsular region of the ovary, while in GCP, the cysts occupy the entire parenchyma of the ovary. It was reported that frequency of abnormally high androstenedione concentrations was higher in the GCP group than in the PCP group. It was shown that ultrasound examination was related to two different patterns of catecholamine metabolism.

A good correlation has been shown between ultrasound diagnoses of polycystic morphology and histopathological criteria for polycystic ovaries by studies examining ovarian tissue obtained at hysterectomy.[7]

Transabdominal ultrasound

One group was among the first to use high-resolution real-time ultrasound to describe polycystic ovaries.[8] Prior to this it was thought that the tiny cysts/follicles of the polycystic ovary could not be detected by ultrasound. The follicles were noted to be 2–6 mm in diameter but their number was neither recorded nor defined.

Ultrasound was used to describe the ovarian appearance in women classified as having polycystic ovarian syndrome rather than to make the diagnosis. Criteria set out by Franks et al.[6] defined a polycystic ovary as one which contains, in one plane at least, 10 follicles (between 2 and 8 mm in diameter) usually arranged peripherally around a dense core of ovarian stroma or scattered throughout an increased amount of stroma. Franks et al.'s criteria have been adopted by many subsequent studies that have used ultrasound scanning to detect polycystic ovaries.

Transvaginal scanning superseded transabdominal scanning and from the early 1990s transvaginal scanning was more in use, especially in infertility clinics. The transvaginal approach provided a more accurate view of the structures of the ovaries.

Ovarian volume

A large study[9] calculated the ovarian volume and ovarian stromal area using 6.5 MHz transvaginal probe. Traditionally (even with transabdominal scan) the ovarian volume has been calculated using the prolate ellipsoid formula ($\pi/6 \times$ maximal longitudinal, anterioposterior and transverse diameters). A large number of different ultrasound formulae with different weightings for the diameters were used to calculate ovarian volume but the consensus view is that until more data are collected and validated the volume of the polycystic ovary should be calculated using the widely accepted prolate ellipsoid.

Internal features of the polycystic ovary

Follicle size and number

Technical aspects: it is now known that it is oocyte-containing follicles that were observed when describing the polycystic ovary, rather than pathological or atretic cystic structures.[5] The early literature often refers to 'cysts' rather than follicles, and the latter are indeed small cysts.

Each ovary should be scanned in longitudinal cross-section from the inner to outer margins in order to count the total number of cysts/follicles. Follicle number should be estimated in two planes of the ovary in order to estimate their size and position. The diameter of follicles is measured as the mean of three diameters. Different studies have described the polycystic ovary with a different number of follicles.

Polycystic ovaries were originally defined as having (in one plane) at least 10 follicles (usually between 2–8 mm) and usually arranged peripherally.[6] Later on it was claimed that the transvaginal definition of the polycystic ovary should require the presence of at least 15 follicles (2–10 mm diameter).[10]

A large study[11] of 214 PCOs performed transvaginal scanning 7 MHz, analysing three different categories of follicle size (2–5 mm, 6–9 mm and 2–9 mm). The mean follicle number per ovary (FNPO) was similar between normal and polycystic ovaries in the 6–9 mm range but significantly higher in the polycystic ovaries in both the 2–5 mm and 2–9 mm ranges. The FNPO of >12 follicles of 2–9 mm gave the best threshold for diagnosis of PCOs. If there is a follicle >10 mm in diameter, the scan is repeated at a time of ovarian quiescence in order to calculate the volume and area.

The consensus definition for a polycystic ovary is one that contains 12 or more follicles of 2–9 mm diameter. This would help to discriminate polycystic ovaries from other causes of multifollicular ovaries.

The multicystic ovary is one in which there are multiple follicles (up to six, usually 4–10 mm in diameter) with normal stromal echogenicity. The term multifollicular is preferred to multicystic and is characteristically seen during puberty.

Appearance of stroma

The increased echodensity of the polycystic ovary is a key histological feature, but the ultrasonographic assessment could be subjective depending on the setting of the ultrasound machine and the patient's body habitus.

The normal stromal echogenicity is said to be less than that of the myometrium. This study showed that the sensitivity and specificity of ovarian stromal echogenicity in the diagnosis of polycystic ovaries were 94% and 90% respectively.[12]

A computer-assisted method concluded that an analysis of the ovarian stromal area is better than quantification of the follicles.[13] The stromal index (mean stromal echogenicity: mean echogenicity of entire ovary) was found to be higher in PCOS. The authors concluded that increased stromal echogenicity was due both to increased stromal volume alongside reduced echogenicity of multiple follicles.[14]

The increased stromal volume was found to be the main cause of ovarian enlargement in polycystic ovaries.[15]

The authors reviewed the evidence for international consensus definitions and concluded that increased stromal echogenicity and stromal volume were specific to PCOS.[5] Three-dimensional and Doppler ultrasound studies may be useful research tools but are not required in the definition of PCOS.

Role of Doppler and 3D ultrasound

Doppler allows assessment of the vascular network within the ovarian stroma. Intra-ovarian stromal blood flow has demonstrated a low resistance index in the stroma of polycystic ovaries.[16]

Three-dimensional ultrasound is a relatively new imaging modality that permits improved spatial awareness, true volumetric calculation and quantitative assessment of vascularity within the defined volume of tissues.

This study[17] highlighted the potential importance of the objective quantification of stromal echogenicity and revealed important differences between women with PCOS who are of normal weight or hyperandrogenic, and their counterparts, supporting the concept that ovarian characteristics may influence or be influenced by the phenotypic expression of the disease.

Complications of PCOS

Complications of PCOS include the following.

- Obesity.
- Type 2 diabetes: the risk is between 10%–20%. Up to 40% will have type 2 diabetes or impaired glucose tolerance by the age of 40. Women with central obesity and a family history remain at the highest risk. A woman presenting with PCOS and with a family history of diabetes must have a regular fasting blood sugar check.
- Hypertension.
- Hypertriglyceridaemia.
- Infertility.
- Miscarriage: miscarriage rates have been quoted as between 30%–60%. Women with high LH levels are at increased risk of miscarriage.
- Increased risk of gestational diabetes during pregnancy.
- Increased risk of myocardial infarction among middle-aged women with PCOS. Two recent studies presented at the Society for Endocrinology 2012 meeting showed PCOS increased the risk of MI tenfold.[20]
- Endometrial cancer: women with amenorrhoea and oligomenorrhoea are associated with anovulation and low levels of progesterone. This unopposed action of oestrogen causes endometrial proliferation, and if untreated, hyperplasia and endometrial carcinoma.
- Sleep apnoea: this is an independent risk factor for cardiovascular disease and should be managed by a specialist in a dedicated sleep apnoea clinic.

Treatment

- **Weight loss**: the more obese a woman is, the worse her endocrine profile will be. Weight reduction improves ovulation and pregnancy rates. The aim should be a BMI between 20–26 kg/m². Refer the patient to a health trainer if available in your area. Advise the patient on a low-carbohydrate and low-fat diet.

- **Metformin**: this works by reducing insulin concentration. Raised insulin concentration causes ovarian stimulation to produce more testosterone. The starting dose should be 500 mg twice a day, increasing to 850 mg twice a day if necessary. The main side effects are gastrointestinal and include abdominal pains, diarrhoea and excessive wind. Metformin therapy should be combined with a diet and exercise programme to achieve the maximised benefit.

- **Combined oral contraceptive pill (COC)**: the most effective pill which works for hyperandrogenic symptoms such as acne and hirsutism is Dianette. This contains cyproterone acetate, which blocks the androgen hormone. If this fails then high-dose cyproterone acetate 50 mg once daily given either in combination with estradiol valerate for 21 days or alone for the first 10 days of the cycle, is very effective. Cyproterone acetate can cause liver toxicity, so liver function tests should be carried

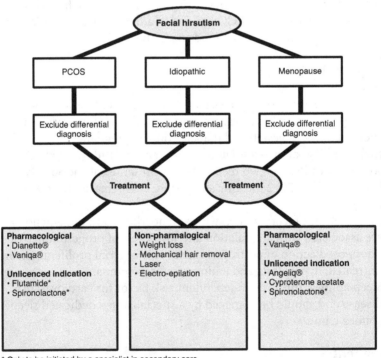

* Only to be initiated by a specialist in secondary care

FIGURE 22.7 Facial hirsutism

out regularly, before starting the therapy and then annually. Yasmin, containing drospirenone combined with ethinyl oestradiol has been shown to be effective. Drospirenone has anti-androgenic activity.

- **For hirsutism**: for facial hirsutism advise mechanical hair removal. Weight loss may be beneficial. Dianette has been shown to be effective. The benefits are short-lived. Spironolactone and cyproterone acetate are unlicensed medications and should not be prescribed. Waxing, laser therapy, electrolysis and bleaching are options (none of these are available on the NHS).

- **Clomiphene**: clomiphene citrate is the first-line therapy for PCOS to induce ovulation. It acts directly on anterior pituitary. It is an anti-oestrogen. Clomiphene is given orally in a dose of 50 mg starting on day 2 of the cycle for 5 days. It is good practice for all cycles to be monitored by ultrasound scans and blood tests. Clomiphene is more useful than metformin alone for women to achieve pregnancy. The cumulative conception rate is 67% after six cycles and the risk of multiple pregnancies is 11%. The findings of a more recent paper suggested that combination therapy was superior to clomiphene therapy.[18] Trials comparing the benefit of combination therapy (metformin plus clomiphene) with clomiphene alone showed a significant benefit with the combined therapy.[19]

- **Gonadotrophin therapy**: gonadotrophins are available in the form of urinary-derived human menopausal gonadotrophins (HMGs). If the patient fails to ovulate with clomiphene, gonadotrophin is the next step. Risk of multiple pregnancy and ovarian hyperstimulation can be reduced by using a low dose of HMG.

- **Ovarian drilling**: ovarian drilling with a diathermy needle can achieve an ovulation rate of up to 90%. This is carried out as a day case under general anaesthetic. Four millimetre holes are placed in each ovary with an ovarian diathermy.

- **In vitro fertilisation**: this is the final option if all the above treatments fail.

KEY POINTS

- Polycystic ovaries occur in 20%–25% of women and are diagnosed by ultrasound scanning.
- The Rotterdam consensus definition provides a helpful framework for the diagnosis and management of PCOS.
- The diagnosis of mild PCOS or even the presence of polycystic ovaries alone should alert the GP to advise women to avoid weight gain, which causes a worsening of the syndrome and greater long-term morbidity.

- Polycystic ovarian syndrome (PCOS) is defined as the presence of two of these: oligomenorrhoea and/or anovulation, hyperandrogenisation and polycystic ovaries.
- Patients requiring fertility treatment should be referred.
- Patients seeking help with obesity can be treated by a GP.
- The GP must do annual blood sugar checks in a patient presenting with PCOS and with a strong family history of diabetes.
- Metformin treatment should be combined with a dietary and exercise regime to achieve the maximum benefit on regulation of menstruation and ovulation.
- Clomiphene is the first-line medical fertility treatment in PCOS.
- Ovarian drilling with a diathermy offers cumulative pregnancy rates of 70%.

Useful websites

For patients

Women's Health Concern is a charitable organisation that helps to educate women on health issues: www.womens-health-concern.org

For GPs

PCOS UK is a multidisciplinary society for healthcare professionals: www.pcos-uk. org.uk

Royal College of Obstetricians and Gynaecologists. Polycystic ovary syndrome, long-term consequences. Green-top guideline 33. London: RCOG; 2003. www.rcog.org.uk/womens-health/clinical-guidance/long-term-consequences-polycystic-ovary-syndrome-green-top-33

References

1 Rotterdam ESHRE/ASRM-Sponsored PCOS Consensus Workshop Group. Revised 2003 consensus on diagnostic criteria and long-term health risks related to polycystic ovary syndrome (PCOS). *Fertil Steril.* 2004; **81**(1): 19–25.
2 Setji TL, Brown AJ. Polycystic ovary syndrome: diagnosis and treatment. *Am J Med.* 2007; **120**(2): 128–32.
3 Rees M, Hope S, Oehler MK. *Problem Solving in Women's Health.* Oxford: Clinical Publishing; 2008.
4 Bates J. *Practical Gynaecological Ultrasound.* Cambridge: Cambridge University Press; 2006.
5 Balen AH, Laven JS, Tan SL, *et al.* Ultrasound assessment of the polycystic ovary: international consensus definitions. *Human Reproduction Update.* 2003; 9(6): 505–14.

6 Franks S, Adams J, Mason H, *et al.* Ovulatory disorders in women with polycystic ovary syndrome. *Clin Obstet Gynaecol.* 1985; **12**(3): 605–32.

7 Saxton DW, Farquhar CM, Rae T, *et al.* Accuracy of ultrasound measurements of female pelvic organs. *Br J Obstet Gynaecol.* 1990; **97**(8): 695–9.

8 Swanson M, Sauerbrei EE, Cooperberg PL. Medical implications of ultrasonically detected polycystic ovaries. *Clin Ultrasound.* 1981; **9**(5): 219–22.

9 Fulghesu AM, Ciampelli M, Belosi C, *et al.* A new ultrasound criterion for the diagnosis of polycystic ovary syndrome: the ovarian stroma/total area ratio. *Fertil Steril.* 2001; 76(2): 326–31. www.ncbi.nlm.nih.gov/pubmed/11476780

10 Fox R, Corrigan E, Thomas PA, *et al.* The diagnosis of polycystic ovaries in women with oligo-amenorrhoea; predictive power of endocrine test. *Clin Endocrinol (Oxf).* 1991; 34: 127–31.

11 Jonard S, Robert Y, Cortet-Rudelli C, *et al.* Ultrasound examination of polycystic ovaries: is it worth counting the follicles? *Hum Reprod.* 2003; 18: 598–603.

12 Pache TD, Wladimiroff JW, Hop WC, *et al.* How to discriminate between normal and polycystic ovaries: transvaginal US study. *Radiology.* 1992; **183**(2): 421–3.

13 Dewailly D. Definition and significance of polycystic ovaries. *Baillieres Clin Obstet Gynaecol.* 1997; **11**(2): 349–68.

14 Buckett WM, Bouzayen R, Watkin KL. Ovarian stromal echogenicity in women with normal and polycystic ovaries. *Hum Reprod.*1999; 14: 618–21.

15 Kyei-Mensah A, Maconochie N, Zaidi J, *et al.* Transvaginal three-dimensional ultrasound: accuracy of follicular volume measurements. *Fertile Steril.* 1996; **65**(2): 371–6.

16 Battagalia C, Artini PG, D' Ambrogio G, *et al.* The role of colour Doppler imaging in the diagnosis of polycystic ovary syndrome. *Am J Obstet Gynecol.* 1995; **172**(1 Pt 1): 108–13.

17 Lam Po M, Johnson I and Fenning N. Three dimensional ultrasound features of the polycystic ovary and the effect of different phenotypic expressions on these parameters. *Human Rep.* 2007; **22**(12): 3116–23.

18 Legro RS, Barnhart HX, Schlaff WD, *et al.* Clomiphene, metformin, or both for infertility in the polycystic ovarian syndrome. *N Engl J Med.* 2007; **356**(6): 551–66.

19 Sinha A, Atiomo W. The role of metformin in the treatment of infertile women with polycystic ovary syndrome. *Obstet Gynecol (Lond).* 2004; 6: 145–51.

20 Robinson S. Polycystic ovary syndrome increases risk of MI 10-fold. *GP Online.* 27 March 2012. Available at: http://m.gponline.com/article/1123698/Polycystic-ovary-syndrome-increases-risk-MI-10-fold (accessed 16 December 2012).

21 Royal College of Obstetricians and Gynaecologists (RCOG). Polycystic ovary syndrome: long–term consequences. Green-top guideline 33. RCOG; 2007. www.rcog.org.uk

23

Endometrial cancer

Prevalence

Endometrial cancer is now the most common gynaecological malignancy in the Western world, having surpassed ovarian cancer over the last 10 years.[1] It is the seventh commonest cancer in women and the most common gynaecological malignancy in the developed world.[2] The incidence is increasing due to a rising level of obesity, diabetes mellitus, an increasing ageing population and the use of oestrogenic drugs, which predispose towards disease onset and progression. Approximately 10% of cancers occur in women less than 50 years of age.[3] Traditionally it is thought that endometrial cancer, due to its earlier recognition, has a better prognosis than the other gynaecological malignancies. To an extent this is true, as it has an overall 5-year survival of ~75%.

Staging and 5-year survival

Endometrial cancer is staged according to the histology and cytology results after surgery. The stage determines the extent of cancer growth in and beyond the uterus. Staging is done after hysterectomy. The grade of endometrial cancer refers to how the cancer cells look under the microscope.

Endometrial cancer staging allows appropriate treatment options. Staging can be based on the TNM or FIGO classification.

FIGO Staging for carcinoma of the endometrium[4]
- **stage 0**: carcinoma in situ
- **stage I**: limited to the body of the uterus
  - **Ia**: no or less than half myometrial invasion
  - **Ib**: invasion equal to or more than half of the myometrium

- **stage II**: cervical stromal involvement
  — endocervical glandular involvement only is stage I
- **stage III**: local or regional spread of the tumour
  — **IIIa**: tumour invades the serosa of the body of the uterus and or adenexae
  — **IIIb**: vaginal or parametrial involvement
  — **IIIc**: pelvic or para-aortic lymphadenopathy
    ¤ **IIIc1**: positive pelvic nodes
    ¤ **IIIc2**: positive para-aortic nodes with or without pelvic nodes
- **stage IV**: Involvement of rectum and or bladder mucosa and or distant metastasis
  — **IVa**: bladder or rectal mucosal involvement
  — **IVb**: distant metastases, malignant ascites, peritoneal involvement

TABLE 23.1 TNM Classification

REGIONAL LYMPH NODES (N)		
TNM	FIGO stages	Surgical-pathologic findings
NX		Regional lymph nodes cannot be assessed
N0		No regional lymph node metastasis
N1	IIIC1	Regional lymph node metastasis to pelvic lymph nodes
N2	IIIC2	Regional lymph node metastasis to para-aortic lymph nodes, with or without positive pelvic lymph nodes
Distant metastasis (M)		
TNM	FIGO stages	Surgical-pathologic findings
M0		No distant metastasis
M1	IVB	Distant metastasis (includes metastasis to inguinal lymph nodes, intraperitoneal disease, or lung, liver, or bone metastases; it excludes metastasis to para-aortic lymph nodes, vagina, pelvic serosa, or adnexa)

The staging for endometrial cancer and its corresponding 5-year survival is shown in Table 23.2.[4]

TABLE 23.2 Staging of endometrial cancer with 5-year survival rate

Stage	I Confined to the uterus	II Involving the cervical stroma	III Local and regional spread: adnexal/vaginal spread, pelvic and para-aortic lymph-nodes	IV Invasion of bowel/bladder mucosa or distant metastasis
5-year survival	85%	75%	45%	25%

Aetiology – risk factors[1]

The risk factors for developing histopathological type I endometrial cancer, which is the most prevalent, relate to endogenous or exogenous exposure to oestrogen. These are:

- obesity
- older age
- diabetes mellitus
- diet high in fat
- early menarche
- late menopause
- nulliparity
- subfertility
- polycystic ovarian syndrome (due to anovulatory cycles)
- oestrogen producing ovarian tumours
- use of tamoxifen: more women are now receiving tamoxifen; this has been shown to prevent breast cancer recurrence, but it is associated with a 3–6-fold increased incidence of endometrial cancer; the risk increases with higher doses and longer duration of usage
- hormone replacement therapy.

A family history of breast, colon and endometrial cancer (all oestrogen dependent) or personal history of breast or colon cancer, also make up predisposing factors in developing endometrial cancer. Hereditary non-polyposis colorectal cancer is one of the commonest cancer family syndromes. There is an estimated 42%–60% lifetime risk of endometrial cancer in women from these families. In these women endometrial cancer often develops before menopause.

Primary care management

The principles of management in primary care should aim to identify those patients at high risk of endometrial cancer and arrange a prompt referral to gynaecological services.

History

1. History of postmenopausal bleeding (PMB).

   This is defined as an episode of bleeding 12 months or more after the last period. It is the most common symptom present, in 75%–80% of patients diagnosed with endometrial cancer. If a patient presents with PMB, enquire:
   - how heavy is the bleeding?
   - when did it start?

- how long does the bleeding last for?
- any history of trauma?
- any relation to sexual intercourse?
- smear status
- drug history: anticoagulants, tamoxifen, levonorgestrel-releasing intrauterine system
- history of taking HRT
- medical or family history.

However, a single episode of PMB will only be due to endometrial cancer in 10% of cases; other explanations could be endometrial polyps, pelvic infection or vaginal trauma due to atrophy. Nevertheless, urgent referral under 2-week referral criteria to secondary services is recommended after an episode of PMB.

Women should be seen in secondary care within 2 weeks to ensure compliance with the 62-day national guideline on cancer treatment times.

The absolute risk of endometrial cancer in non-users of hormone replacement therapy who present with PMB ranges from 5.7% to 11.5%.[5]

2. History of menstrual disturbance: irregular cycles or intermenstrual bleeding.
3. Postmenopausal discharge: brownish or blood-stained?
4. History of lower urinary tract symptoms – *may be a pointer towards the spread of disease.*
5. Any alteration in bowel habits – *may be a pointer towards the spread of disease.*
6. Pelvic pain: this normally is the case when the tumour has spread to adjacent structures such as bowel or bladder.
7. Past medical history of breast or colorectal cancer or tamoxifen therapy.
8. Enquire about the family history of breast, endometrial and colorectal status.
9. History of medical co-morbidities such as obesity, diabetes and related disorders as this might be relevant to further treatment if cancer is confirmed, e.g. treatment modality, surgery versus radiotherapy.

Examination

General physical

- Record body mass index as this is relevant as a risk factor and to further management.
- Blood pressure.
- Signs of anaemia (secondary to PMB).

Physical examination

This should include abdominal and pelvic examination. Check for any organomegaly, e.g. hepatomegaly due to liver metastasis.

Pelvic examination

A bimanual pelvic and per speculum examination must be performed.

- Fixed, enlarged uterus on bimanual palpation.
- Check for any local lesion with speculum examination (e.g. cervical polyp or malignant lesion), discharge and any atrophic changes.
- Perform a cervical smear if patient is due for one.

Investigations

A full blood count to check for anaemia should be performed. If an urgent 2-week referral is made, the transvaginal ultrasonography (TVUS) takes place in secondary care.

Management of endometrial cancer

Modern management is best delivered as part of a one-stop service. Using this approach, women with PMB can be dealt with efficiently on an outpatient basis, with only one visit. The aim is to provide a diagnosis and a management plan all at the same time. All women will need a TVUS and an endometrial biopsy. Women with PMB who have endometrial cancer can then be fast-tracked to the MDT (multidisciplinary team).

The majority of hospitals provide a one-stop postmenopausal clinic; however the correct primary diagnostic tool remains undecided. Some gynaecologists favour TVUS, while others favour hysteroscopy. Data from a randomised controlled trial showed that more patients preferred TVUS to hysteroscopy.[6] Incidental ovarian or adnexal pathologies may be picked up by completing an ultrasound.

Transvaginal ultrasound: a high frequency transducer (6–7.5 MHz) is placed in close proximity to the pelvic organs. Abdominal probes are used to visualise pelvic masses that extend beyond the focal length of the vaginal probe (approximately 10 cm). With TVUS an accurate diagnosis of endometrial polyp, endometrial hyperplasia and endometrial cancer can be made.

Hysteroscopy: hysteroscopy allows direct inspection of endometrial cavity and endocervical canal as well as targeted biopsy and removal of polyps. An outpatient procedure using a 30-degree telescope is the preferred choice unless the woman has a strong preference for a general anaesthetic. In a study of 276 patients who underwent both hysteroscopy and dilation and curettage (D&C), hysteroscopy yielded more information in 44 patients while D&C gave information in 9 patients only.[7] A hysteroscopy should be performed first line in women with recurrent postmenopausal bleed, regardless of endometrial thickness.

Magnetic resonance imaging (MRI): hysteroscopy and TVUS do not give enough information about cervical or deep myometrial invasion. MRI provides this information and also highlights enlarged pelvic lymph nodes. CT scan is reserved for cases where there is a suspicion of distant metastasis.

Endometrial biopsy: endometrial biopsy provides histological confirmation of pathology. The 2007 NICE guidance on heavy menstrual bleeding has provided clear guidance as to who should be referred to secondary services for endometrial biopsy. This is often relevant to women 40–50 years of age.[17]

- Women 45 years old presenting with a menstrual disturbance – e.g. menorrhagia, intermenstrual bleeding (IMB) – should be investigated further with ultrasound pelvis and endometrial biopsy.
- Women over 40 years old, with failed medical therapy or symptoms of intermenstrual bleeding or abnormal physical findings on examination, should be further investigated as above.
- Women over 40 years of age with regular heavy periods and no other symptoms (e.g. IMB) can have a trial of medical therapy (e.g. antifibrinolytics or Mirena coil) prior to further investigation or referral.
- For women taking tamoxifen, hysteroscopy and endometrial biopsy are usually recommended as first-line investigations since there is no agreed cut-off for endometrial thickness in these patients.

Cut-off values for endometrial thickness on TVUS in women with PMB (these values help to identify those at higher risk of endometrial cancer who require further investigations):[8]

Endometrial thickness ≤ 3 mm.
- In women who:
  — have never used HRT
  — have not used any form of HRT for one year or more
  — are taking continuous combined HRT.
- No further action need to be taken.
- If symptoms recur, take further action.

Endometrial thickness ≤ 5 mm.
- For women on sequential combined HRT therapy presenting with unscheduled bleeding, further investigations should be carried out.

Dilatation and curettage (D&C): this has largely been superseded by aspiration curettage, performed either during hysteroscopy or using an endometrial sampling device.

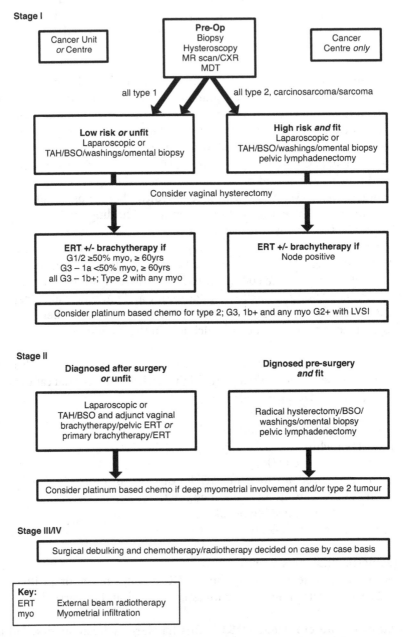

FIGURE 23.1 Algorithm for management of patients with endometrial cancer

Principles of management for confirmed endometrial cancer in secondary care

This depends upon the stage the cancer is diagnosed and is managed by a team of gynae-oncologists, who together with a histopathologist, radiologist and clinical oncologist constitute the Gynae-Oncology Multi-Disciplinary Meeting. Although staging is surgico-pathological (i.e. obtained after an operation), pre-operative investigations often point towards the right direction, so that the right treatment modality (surgery or chemo-radiotherapy) can be chosen.

Pre-operative investigations

- Chest radiograph to exclude lung metastasis.
- MRI pelvis for radiological staging of the tumour.
- Endometrial biopsy for the grade of the tumour.
- Full blood count to exclude anaemia and U+E and LFT depending on additional co-morbidities.

Treatment

If hysteroscopy is negative and histology benign, the patient may be reassured. Consider referral for reinvestigations after 6 months if symptoms reoccur or persist.

Women with confirmed malignancy should be referred to a gynaecology-oncology specialist. Surgery is the first-line treatment. Radiotherapy can be given to those who are not fit enough to have surgery and can be used postoperatively to reduce the risk of recurrence.

Women with simple or complex hyperplasia with no atypical cells on cytology can be managed conservatively.

Surgery

With regard to treatment, for early stage disease (stages I and II), surgery is the primary form of treatment, consisting of a total abdominal hysterectomy, bilateral salpingo-oophorectomy +/– pelvic/para-aortic lymphadenectomy.

Surgery is commonly performed abdominally through a Pfannenstiel incision together with peritoneal washings for cytological staging. Surgery for suspected grade 1 FIGO stage 1A disease may be performed at cancer units – usually the local district general hospital – but the surgery for higher grade and advanced stage should be carried out by a specialist multidisciplinary team at a cancer centre. Minimal access techniques may be used for endometrial cancer surgery including laparoscopic hysterectomy, which may reduce postoperative morbidity compared with open access surgery. Potential benefits are less pain, earlier mobilisation, less hospital stay (*will make the commissioners happy*), and reduced risk of thromboembolism.[9,10] Survival rate and disease-free survival appear to be compatible with conventional open surgery.[11] The role of lymphadenectomy in endometrial cancer treatment remains unclear. Removal of lymph nodes enables adequate staging which may guide adjuvant therapy.

Postoperative pelvic radiotherapy

Pelvic radiotherapy has been shown to significantly reduce the risk of recurrence of stage 1 endometrial cancer within the pelvis but with no demonstrable effect on survival rate.[12] External beam pelvic radiotherapy has demonstrated an increase in survival according to a Cochrane review meta-analysis.[13]

Medical therapy

Hormonal treatment may be beneficial for palliative control of symptoms in patients with advanced stage disease or those who are not fit for surgery. The current evidence does not support the use of progestogens as primary treatment of endometrial cancer.[13] Medroxyprogesterone acetate may be used starting twice weekly for 3 months, followed by a maintenance dose of once weekly in a dose of 500 mg. Mirena coil has also been shown to be beneficial in treating endometrial cancer.[14]

Follow-up – recurrence

All patients are followed up in secondary care for a period of 5 years. In a rather simplified approach, their management involves follow-up appointments with the gynae-oncologists (who check for symptoms suggesting recurrence), alternating with the clinical oncologists (who manage side effects of chemo-radiotherapy).

Repeat postmenopausal bleeding or a mass on the vault identified on speculum examination, should prompt an urgent referral.

KEY POINTS

- Endometrial cancer is the most common gynaecological malignancy in the developed world.
- The incidence is rising due to increasing levels of obesity, diabetes and use of HRT.
- One-stop clinics provide the early assessment and early diagnosis.
- Postmenopausal bleeding is the hallmark symptom.
- Investigations include assessment of endometrial thickness, hysteroscopy and endometrial biopsy.
- All patients with PMB should be referred under a 2-week pathway.
- Total hysterectomy and bilateral salpingo-oophorectomy remains the mainstay of treatment.

- Adjuvant therapy with chemotherapy, radiotherapy or hormonal therapy is considered in more advanced or high-risk disease.

Useful websites

For patients – helplines

Cancer Advice – website designed to inform patients concerning the present state of knowledge of particular cancers and to highlight modern aspects of treatment: www.canceradvice.co.uk/uterine-cancer

Macmillan Cancer Support www.macmillan.org.uk

Maggie's Centres – charity organisation that provides help with information, benefits advice, psychological support: www.maggiescentres.org

Patient UK – source of health and disease information for patients: www.patient.co.uk

For GPs

FIGO staging system for endometrial cancer: added benefits of MR imaging: www.ncbi.nlm.nih.gov/pubmed/22236905

Investigation of postmenopausal bleeding, SIGN Publication No. 61: www.sign.ac.uk/guidelines/fulltext/61/index.html

NICE. Referral for suspected cancer (CG27): www.nice.org.uk/CG027

Postmenopausal bleeding, Map of Medicine: www.mapofmedicine.com

References

1 Shaw R. *Carcinoma of the Ovary and Fallopian Tube in Gynaecology.* 4th edition. Edinburgh: Elsevier; 2011. Chapter 39.

2 Ferlay J, Bray F, Pisani P, *et al.* GLOBOCAN 2002: cancer incidence, mortality and prevalence worldwide. IARC CancerBase no 5, version 2.0. Lyon: IARC Press; 2004.

3 Calle EE, Rodriguez C, Walker-Thurmond K, *et al.* Overweight, obesity and mortality from cancer in a prospectively studied cohort of US adults. *N Eng J Med.* 2003; 348: 1625–38.

4 Pecorelli S. Revised FIGO staging for carcinoma of the vulva, cervix and endometrium. *Int J Gynecol Obstet.* 2009; 105: 103–4.

5 Gredmark T, Kvint S, Havel G, *et al.* Histopathological findings in women with postmenopausal bleeding. *Br J Obstet Gynaecol.* 1995; 102: 133–6.

6 Timmerman D, Deprest J, Bourne T, *et al.* A randomised trial on the use of ultrasound or office hysteroscopy for endometrial assessment in postmenopausal patients with breast cancer who were treated with tamoxifen. *Am J Obstet Gynecol.* 1998; 179: 62–70.

7 Gimpleson R, Rappold H. A comparative study between panoramic hysteroscopy with directed biopsies and dilatation and curettage. *Am J Obstet Gynecol.* 1988; 158: 489–92.

8 Scottish Intercollegiate Guidelines Network. Investigation of post-menopausal bleeding. SIGN guideline 61. Edinburgh: SIGN; 2012. www.sign.ac.uk/pdf/sign61.pdf

9 Eltabbakh GH, Shamonki MI, Moody JM, *et al.* Hysterectomy for obese women with endometrial cancer: laparoscopy or laparotomy? *Gynecol Oncol.* 2000; 78: 329–35.

10 Scribner J, Dennis R, Walker JL, *et al.* Surgical management of early-stage endometrial cancer in the elderly: is laparoscopy feasible? *Gynecol Oncol.* 2001; 83: 563–8.

11 Eltabbakh GH. Analysis of survival after laparoscopy in women with endometrial carcinoma. *Cancer.* 2002; 95: 1894–1901.

12 Scholten AN, Van Putten WLJ, Beerman H, *et al.* Postoperative radiotherapy for stage 1 endometrial carcinoma: long term outcome of the randomised PORTEC trial with central pathology review. *Int J Radiation Oncology Biol Phys.* 2005; 63: 834–8.

13 Martin-Hirsch PL, Jarvis GG, Kitchener HC, *et al.* Progestogens for endometrial cancer. Cochrane Database Syst Rev. 1999; 4: CD001040.

14 Giannopoulos T, Butler-Manuel SA, Tailor A. Levonorgestrel releasing intrauterine system LNG-IUS as a therapy for endometrial carcinoma. *Gynecol Oncol.* 2004; 95: 762–4.

15 ASTEC Study Group, Kitchener H, Swart AM, *et al.* Efficacy of systematic pelvic lymphadenectomy in endometrial cancer. *Lancet.* 2009; **373**(9658): 125–36.

16 ASTEC/EN.5 Study Group, Blake P, Swart AM, *et al.* Adjuvant external beam radiotherapy in the treatment of endometrial cancer. *Lancet.* 2009; **373**(9658): 137–46.

17 National Institute for Health and Clinical Excellence. Heavy menstrual bleeding: NICE guideline 44. London: NIHCE; 2007. www.nice.org.uk/CG044

24

Uterine fibroids

> **DEFINITION**
>
> Fibroids are benign tumours arising from the myometrium of the uterus affecting premenopausal women and often associated with significant morbidity. They are sometimes known as uterine myomas, fibromyomas, leiomyoma or leiomyomata. Fibroids are made up of muscle and fibrous tissue and can vary in size.

Prevalence

Many women are unaware that they have fibroids, as they are asymptomatic. They are diagnosed by chance during a routine pelvic examination or an ultrasound scan of the pelvis. Data regarding their prevalence is limited. In general it can be said that fibroids usually develop during a woman's reproductive years from approximately 16–50 years of age. Fibroids do not occur in pre-pubertal girls.[1] After puberty, the prevalence increases until the menopause stage.[1] The prevalence of symptomatic fibroids is low in women younger than 30 years of age.[1]

In a study of 12 500 younger women undergoing a routine prenatal ultrasound, the prevalence of fibroids was 1.5%.[2]

The prevalence of fibroids is higher in African-Caribbean women than in Caucasian women. In a US study of 1364 women of the age group 35–49 years, approximately 60% of African-Caribbean women had detectable fibroid by 35 years of age, which increased to 80% by 49 years of age.[3]

Aetiology

The aetiology of fibroids is not understood completely. The risk factors are outlined in the following.

- Increasing age: The prevalence varies with age, with an increase in late reproductive years, affecting more than 30% of women aged 40–60 years.[5]
- Puberty: the risk of fibroids is slightly increased in women who experience early menarche, although this is not statistically significant.[6] Early onset of menarche may cause an increased chance of gene mutation in controlling myometrial proliferation.[7]
- Parity: several studies have shown an inverse relationship between parity and risk of fibroids.[6,8] An explanation of this finding is that pregnancy reduces the time of exposure to unopposed oestrogens.[4]
- Pregnancy: epidemiological data shows that pregnancy is associated with reduced risk of fibroids. This is due to the protective effect of postpartum involution of the uterus.[9]
- Menopause: a reduced risk in menopause could be due to shrinkage of fibroid in the absence of hormonal stimulus.[4,6]
- Race: African-Caribbean women are more likely to develop fibroids than Caucasian women, and at an early age. The fibroids tend to be larger and more symptomatic.[3,5]
- Obesity: fibroids are 2–3 times more common in obese women. In a prospective study from Great Britain, the risk of fibroid increased approximately 21% for each 10 kg increase in body weight.[4] The association between obesity and increased risk of fibroid may be related to hormonal factors associated with obesity. This is thought to be due to the conversion of circulating adrenal androgens to oestrone by excessive adipose tissue.
- Eating habits: there is evidence to suggest that a diet rich in green vegetables decreases the risk, and excessive intake of beef and ham is associated with increased risk.[10] There is no evidence that a change in diet has any impact on the patient's symptoms once the diagnosis is made.
- Exercise: an increased exercise is associated with relative leanness and in turn with reduced conversion of androgens to oestrogens in adipose tissue.[11]
- Smoking: smoking appears to reduce the risk of fibroid formation and growth. This is thought to be due to reduction in the circulating sex hormone-binding globulin (SHBG), which is a direct result of the effect of smoking on liver enzymes. As a result there is an increase in the level of free oestrogens, which has a mitogenic effect on fibroids.[4,6,11]
- Hormonal method of contraception: the evidence is conflicting and

is considered insignificant by some experts.[1] Some studies found no increase in association between the occurrence of fibroid and oral contraceptives,[6] while others have reported a significant reduction in the risk of fibroid and oral contraceptive use.[4]

- Hormone replacement therapy (HRT): fibroids shrink after menopause but the use of HRT may prevent this shrinkage and may even stimulate growth.[12]
- Tamoxifen: the in vivo effect of tamoxifen in both pre- and postmenopausal women at a dosage level used for patients with breast cancer, is either to stimulate the growth of fibroid or to exert no effect.[13]
- Theory of initiation: one hypothesis states an increase in mitotic rate caused by increased level of oestrogens and progestogens resulting in formation of myoma by increasing the likelihood of somatic mutation.[14]
- Genetic factors: genetic and hereditary factors are being considered and several epidemiological studies indicate genetic influence for early onset fibroid. Chromosomal abnormalities are present in nearly 50% of fibroids and mutations in the MED12 gene have been documented in 70% of fibroids. It is well established that first-degree relatives have a 2.5-fold increased risk and there can be nearly a 6-fold increased risk in early onset cases.[15]

Classification

Fibroids are often classified as:
- Intramural: they are the most common fibroids and develop within the lining of the uterus, tending to expand inwards and increasing the size of the uterus, resulting in heavy and prolonged bleeding, pelvic pain, back pain and a generalised feeling of pressure.
- Submucosal: they are just under the lining of the uterus. They are the least common fibroids but tend to cause the most problems. Even a small submucosal fibroid can cause heavy and prolonged bleeding. Submucosal fibroids are further classified as type O, I, II, depending on how much they project into the uterine cavity.
- Subserosal: they develop under the outside covering of the uterus and expand outwards, giving the uterus a knobby appearance. They typically do not affect the menstrual flow but can cause back pains, pelvic pains and a pressure feeling.
- Pedunculated: if on a long stalk inside the uterine cavity or on the outside of the uterus.
- Rarely fibroids are located in the round ligament, broad ligament or the uterosacral ligament of the uterus.

Primary care management

History

There are often no symptoms present and fibroids are detected during routine pelvic examination. Symptoms depend on the size, location and number of fibroids. Enquire about the history of:

- periods: duration, whether heavy with clots, any associated pain/abdominal discomfort
- any intermenstrual bleed (IMB) – *for a woman presenting with abnormal uterine bleeding, it is important to exclude underlying endometrial pathology*
- acute haemorrhage – *a woman presenting with acute haemorrhage related to fibroid (rare but life-threatening condition) must be admitted*
- any associated back pain/discomfort
- pelvic pain and/or pressure feeling – *pelvic pain is rare with fibroids and it usually signifies degeneration, torsion or adenomyosis*[23]
- sensation of fullness in the lower abdomen
- associated urinary symptoms: frequency, pressure on bladder causing urgency or retention
- bowel symptoms: constipation, bloated feeling or painful defecation
- painful intercourse (dyspareunia)
- infertility
- past obstetric history: any miscarriages, premature labour, difficult labour.

Examination

Look for signs of anaemia.

- Per abdominal examination: a palpable abdominal mass may be felt. *Generally, fibroids the size of a grapefruit or bigger can be felt by the patient and are easily palpable on pelvic examination.*
- A pelvic examination may be difficult if patient is obese. All patients presenting with symptoms suggestive of fibroids must have a bimanual pelvic examination to assess the size, position and mobility of the uterus.
- A per speculum examination must be carried out to assess the cervix. This could be an opportunity for a smear if indicated.

Differential diagnosis:

- endometrial polyp
- endometriosis
- endometrial cancer
- ovarian tumour
- uterine sarcoma

- pregnancy
- appendix abscess
- diverticular abscess
- tubo-ovarian abscess.

Investigations

- Full blood count (FBC) and serum ferritin to exclude anaemia.
- Pregnancy test if clinically indicated.
- Transvaginal ultrasound scan (TVS). This is a more reliable investigation than abdominal ultrasound in assessing the fibroids, especially in obese patients. The cost-effective aspect of TVS has made it the preferred first line investigation in patients with suspected fibroids. *This investigation is available to GPs as well.*
- MRI: MRI is a costly but powerful tool that is useful in establishing the exact position, characteristics and number of fibroids. MRI is useful in diagnosing pedunculated fibroids that can be confused as an adnexal mass.
- Endometrial sampling: indicated if history of abnormal uterine bleeding.
- Hysteroscopy with biopsy: indicated for assessment of abnormal uterine bleeding.

Management

Primary care management

- Simple analgesia, non-steroidal anti-inflammatories (NSAIDs), oral contraceptives to reduce the pain and bleeding.
- Iron supplements if patient is anaemic. Iron preparations are available over the counter, though it may be cheaper for the patient if they pay a prescription charge.
- Simple health promotion advice regarding healthy eating, increasing exercise. This may not regress the size of the fibroid but will be helpful in case surgery is needed.
- Tranexamic acid: an antifibrinolytic agent to reduce menorrhagia.
- Combined oral contraceptive pill to reduce bleeding and if the patient requires contraception. They are not effective in reducing the size of the fibroids.
- Levonorgestrel intrauterine system (IUS) to reduce menstrual blood-flow. The most common side effect is spontaneous expulsion in patients with fibroids. There is insufficient evidence that they reduce the size of the fibroids.
- Danazol: danazol reduces menorrhagia by suppressing gonadotrophin secretion and ovarian function. It is used rarely because of its side effects.

- Gonadotrophin-releasing hormone (GnRH) analogues: these cause reduction in the size of fibroids by decreasing circulating oestrogen. They are associated with significant side effects including menopausal symptoms and osteoporosis in long-term use. They are mainly used preoperatively to shrink the size of fibroid. They provide an alternative for women who have contraindications to surgery or who do not wish to undergo surgery. Once therapy is stopped, fibroids tend to grow back.

Surgery

- Hysterectomy: for women who have completed their family, hysterectomy is the most effective treatment for heavy uterine bleeding.[16] It is also indicated in patients who have failed to respond to medical management. Laparotomy is indicated with preservation of ovaries if the fibroids are large.[17] If they are small, vaginal route is the treatment of choice. NICE recommends that laparoscopic techniques for hysterectomy are safe and effective. There is, however, a higher risk of urinary tract injury and of severe bleeding as compared to open surgery.[18] When considering hysterectomy for menorrhagia attributed to fibroids, other causes must be ruled out. Endometrial biopsy should be considered to exclude endometrial lesions. Hysterectomy does not offer cure for symptoms of incontinence in the presence of fibroids.
- Uterine artery embolisation (UAE): UAE is safe and effective for women who may wish to have children in future.[19] The procedure can significantly alleviate pain and menstrual blood flow and pressure effects from fibroids. Complications include adverse reactions to the contrast media, haematoma, thrombosis or pseudo-aneurysm. UAE is a good alternative to hysterectomy.[16] The HOPEFUL trial showed that 23% of women required further intervention following UAE at a mean follow-up of 4.6 years.[20] There is evidence to suggest that UAE is associated with spontaneous abortion, pre-term delivery and postpartum haemorrhage.[20]
- Myomectomy: laparoscopic myomectomy is the treatment option for symptomatic women with subserous fibroids who wish to maintain their fertility.[21] There is a small risk of excessive bleeding, requiring hysterectomy at the time of operation.[21] Women should be counselled about the risks of requiring a hysterectomy at the time of a planned myomectomy. There is a 15% recurrence rate for fibroids and 10% of women undergoing a myomectomy will eventually require hysterectomy within 5–10 years.
- Endometrial ablation: endometrial ablation is suitable for those with menstrual bleeding problems.

Fibroid and uterine leiomyosarcomas: uterine sarcoma is a rare gynae-cologic malignancy, occurring in 1.7 per 100 000 women over the age of 20 years.[22] A uterine mass increasing in size in a postmenopausal woman suggests a leiomyosarcoma. There is currently no evidence to substantiate performing a hysterectomy or myomectomy for an asymptomatic leiomy-oma for the sole purpose of alleviating the concern that it may be malignant.

Fibroids in menopause: fibroids usually shrink to about half their original size after menopause. Therefore HRT can cause growth of fibroid in post-menopausal women. Postmenopausal bleeding and pain in women with fibroids should be investigated in the same way as in women without fibroids.

Fibroids and pregnancy: the complications depend upon the size, number and location of the myomas. Fibroids located in the lower uterine segment may increase the likelihood of foetal malpresentation, caesarean section and postpartum haemorrhage. Large fibroids defined as greater than 20 cm in diameter are more likely to cause abruption and abdominal pain.[24] Myomectomy should not be performed in pregnant women because of increased risk of uncontrolled bleeding.[25]

Complications of fibroids

Complications of fibroids include:

- iron deficiency anaemia
- torsion of pedunculated fibroid
- bladder frequency
- constipation
- infertility
- malignancy: the malignant version is extremely uncommon and is called leiomyosarcoma
- in pregnancy: miscarriage, red degeneration, premature labour, postpartum haemorrhage, foetal malpresentation.

KEY POINTS

- Fibroids are the most common benign tumours and are often asymptomatic.
- Fibroids are more common in African-Caribbean women than in Caucasians.
- Most common symptoms are heavy painful periods, abdominal discomfort, urinary frequency and painful defecation.
- During pregnancy, fibroids may be the cause of miscarriage, premature labour and malpresentation of foetus.
- Fibroids are easy to diagnose by ultrasound scan. Transvaginal scan is more reliable than abdominal scan.

- Medical treatment should be tailored to the needs of the woman presenting with fibroids.
- Iron supplements should be given to anaemic patients.
- Although the long-term response to danazol is poor, it may offer an advantage in reducing menorrhagia.
- Hormone replacement therapy (HRT) should not be used to treat fibroids as it is not effective in reducing uterine fibroid size.
- Gonadotrophin-releasing hormone analogue (GnRH) treatment reduces fibroid size but unpleasant side effects and a reduction in bone mineral density limits its sole use to 6 months.
- Myomectomy is an option for women who wish to preserve their uterus, but the patient should be counselled regarding the risk of requiring a hysterectomy.
- Uterine artery embolisation is a safe and effective radiological technique used in the management of symptomatic fibroid.
- Hysterectomy is the treatment of choice in women who are symptomatic and have completed their family.

Useful websites

For patients – helplines

Fibroids – diagnosis, NHS Choices: www.nhs.uk/conditions/fibroids/pages/diagnosis.aspx

For GPs

NICE. Heavy menstrual bleeding (CG44): http://guidance.nice.org.uk/CG44

Lumsden MA. Modern management of fibroids. *Obstet Gynaecol Reprod.* 2010; 20: 82–6.

References

1 Parker WH. Etiology, symptomatology and diagnosis of uterine myomas. *Fertil Steril.* 2007; **87**(4): 725–36.
2 Cooper NP, Okolo S. Fibroids in pregnancy: common but poorly understood. *Obstet Gynecol Surv.* 2005; **60**(2): 132–8.
3 Day Baird D, Dunson DB, Hill MC, *et al.* High cumulative incidence of uterine leiomyoma in black and white women: ultrasound evidence. *Am J Obstet Gynecol.* 2003; **188**(1): 100–7.
4 Ross RK, Pike MC, Vessey MP, *et al.* Risk factors for uterine fibroids: reduced risk associated with oral contraceptives. *BMJ Clinical Research Edition.* 1986; 293: 359–62.
5 Marshall LM, Spiegelman D, Barbieri RL, *et al.* Variation in the incidence of

uterine leiomyoma among premenopausal women by age. *Obstet Gynaecol.* 1997; **90**(6): 967–73.

6   Samadi AR, Lee NC, Flanders WD, *et al.* Risk factors for self-reported uterine fibroids: a case-control study. *Am J Public Health.* 1996; **86**(6): 856–62.

7   Marshall LM, Spiegelman D, Goldman MB, *et al.* A prospective study of reproductive factors and oral contraceptive use in relation to the risk of uterine leiomyomata. *Fertil Steril.* 1998a; 70: 432–9.

8   Lumbiganon P, Rugpao S, Phandhu-fung S, *et al.* Protective effect of depot-medroxyprogesterone acetate on surgically treated uterine leiomyoma: a multicentre case-control study. *Br J Obstet Gynaecol.* 1996; **103**(9): 909–14.

9   Day B, Donna D, David D. Why is parity protective for uterine fibroids? *Epidemiology.* 2003; **14**(2): 247–50.

10 Chiaffarino F, Parazzini F, La Vecchia C, *et al.* Diet and uterine myomas. *Obstet Gynaecol.* 1999; **94**(3): 395–8.

11 Wyshak G, Frisch RE, Albright NL, *et al.* Lower prevalence of benign diseases of the breast and benign tumours of the reproductive system among former college athletes compared to non-athletes. *Br J Cancer.* 1986; **54**(5): 841–5.

12 Romieu I, Walker AM, Jick S. Determinants of uterine fibroids. *Post Market Surveil.* 1991; 5: 119–33.

13 Kang J, Baxi L, Heller D. Tamoxifen induced growth of leiomyoma: a case report. *J Reprod Med.* 1996; **41**(2): 119–20.

14 Rein MS. Advances in uterine leiomyoma research: the progressive progesterone hypothesis. *Environ Health Perspect.* 2000; **108**(Suppl 5): 791–3.

15 Markowski DN, Bartnitzke S, Loning T, *et al.* MED12 mutations in uterine fibroids: their relationship to cytogenetics subgroups. *Int J Cancer.* 2012; **131**(7): 1528–36.

16 Al-Mahrizi S, Tulandi T. Treatment of uterine fibroids for abnormal uterine bleeding: myomectomy and uterine artery embolization. *Best Pract Res Clin Obstet Gynaecol.* 2007; **21**(6): 995–1005.

17 McPherson K, Metcalfe MA, Herbert A, *et al.* Severe complications of hysterectomy: the VALUE study. *BJOG.* 2004; **111**(7): 688–94.

18 National Institute for Health and Clinical Excellence. Laparoscopic Techniques for Hysterectomy: NICE Technology Appraisal IPG239 London: NIHCE; 2007. www.nice.org.uk/guidance/index.jsp?action=byId&o=11045

19 National Institute for Health and Clinical Excellence. Uterine Artery Embolisation for Fibroids: NICE Interventional Procedure Guidance 367. London: NIHCE; 2010. http://publications.nice.org.uk/uterine-artery-embolisation-for-fibroids-ipg367

20 Dutton S, Hirst A, McPherson K, *et al.* A UK multicentre retrospective cohort study comparing hysterectomy and uterine artery embolisation for the treatment of symptomatic uterine fibroids (HOPEFUL study): main results on medium-term safety and efficacy. *BJOG.* 2007; **114**(11): 1340–51.

21 Agdi M, Tulandi T. Endoscopic management of uterine fibroids. *Best Pract Res Clin Obstet Gynaecol.* 2008; **24**(4): 707–16.

22 DiSaia PJ, Creasman WT. *Clinical Gynecologic Oncology.* 6th ed. St Louis: C.V. Mosby; 2001.

23 Lumsden MA, Wallace EM. Clinical presentation of uterine fibroids. *Baillieres Clin Obstet Gynaecol.* 1998; 12: 177–95.

24 Exacoustos C, Rosati R. Ultrasound diagnosis of uterine myomas and complications in pregnancy. *Obstet Gynecol.* 1993; **82**(5): 97–101.

25 Burton C, Grimes DA, March CM. Surgical management of leiomyomata during pregnancy. *Obstet Gynecol.* 1989; 74: 707–9.

25

Ovarian cancer

Prevalence

Ovarian cancer is the fifth most common cancer in women after breast, colorectal, lung and uterine[1] and the second most common gynaecological cancer in the UK after uterine. Each year in the UK about 6700 new cases are diagnosed. Due to its late presentation its prognosis is worse than the other gynaecological cancers and for this reason a high clinical index of suspicion and prompt referral is essential. Approximately 4300 women die from ovarian cancer each year which makes it the leading cause of death in gynaecological cancers.[1] It accounts for 6% of all cancer deaths in women.[1] This is due to the fact that 75% of women present with advanced stage 3C and 4 disease.[2]

Epidemiology

In the UK, there are approximately 7000 cases of ovarian cancer per year. The majority of women present after the menopause (peak age: 50–70) with an overall lifetime risk of 1 in 48.

Approximately 6700 new cases were diagnosed every year in United Kingdom between 2004 and 2007 accounting for approximately 1 in 20 cases of cancer in women.[3]

About three quarters present with extra-ovarian disease (stages III & IV) and hence the overall 5-year survival is 40%.

Risk factors

Risk factors for ovarian cancer include conditions that increase the number of ovulatory cycles in the lifetime of a woman.

Proven increased risks:
- early menarche
- late menopause
- nulliparity
- long-term hormone replacement therapy (HRT)
- endometriosis
- BRCA1/2 carriers
- strong family history: features such as young age, multiple cancers of the same site and multiple family members affected suggest an underlying cancer syndrome such as hereditary breast and ovarian cancer (HBOC) syndrome, caused by mutations in the BECA1 and BRCA2 genes
- Lynch type 2 hereditary cancer.

Possible increased risks:
- obesity
- smoking
- fertility treatment.

Risk of ovarian cancer increases with age, being most prevalent at 60–75 years.

Histology

Ovarian cancer is classified by histology:
- Epithelial ovarian cancer: serous, mucinous, clear cell and endometroid.
- Germ cell tumours: dysgerminoma, choriocarcinoma and immature teratoma.
- Sex cord stromal tumours: Sertoli-Leydig cell tumours and malignant granulosa cell tumour.

Around 90% of ovarian cancers are epithelial in origin, with the rest consisting of germ cell and sex cord tumours. Epithelial cell origin tumours are the most malignant tumours and usually present in postmenopausal women, whereas the germ cell and stromal types often present at a younger age group.

There are ovarian tumours of a homogenous nature called borderline ovarian cancer. The prognosis for these tumours is much better than for typical epithelial ovarian cancers. They often occur in younger women and as stage 1 tumours.

Staging

It is worth remembering that despite pre-operative imaging giving us some idea, ovarian cancer staging is surgico-pathological; in other words it is only after the surgical removal of the tumour that accurate staging is obtained.

Staging of ovarian cancer is classified according to the International Federation of Gynecology and Obstetrics (FIGO) guidelines – *see* Table 25.1.[2]

TABLE 25.1 FIGO classification of ovarian cancer

	STAGE	DISEASE
Stage1	1A	Limited to one ovary with capsule intact, no ascites
Tumour confined to	1B	Limited to both ovaries with capsules intact, no ascites
the ovaries	1C	Stage 1A or 1B but disease on surface of one or both ovaries, or capsule rupture or malignant cells in ascites or peritoneal washing
Stage 2	2A	Extension or metastasis to the uterus or fallopian tubes
Tumour confined to	2B	Extension or metastasis to other pelvic organs
the pelvis	2C	Stage 1A or 2B with disease on one or both ovaries, or capsule rupture, or malignant cells in ascites or peritoneal washing
Stage 3	3A	Microscopic seeding of tumour on the abdominal peritoneal surfaces or omentum
Tumour confined to the abdomen	3B	Macroscopic metastasis on the abdominal peritoneal surfaces or omentum <2 cm in diameter
	3C	Macroscopic metastasis on the abdominal peritoneal surfaces or omentum >2 cm in diameter or positive retroperitoneal or inguinal lymph nodes
Stage 4	4	Positive cytology on pleural effusion, parenchymal liver metastasis or umbilical metastasis or other extra-abdominal sites
Distant spread outside of the abdomen		

TABLE 25.2 Ovarian cancer staging and 5-year survival

Stage	I Confined to the ovaries	II Involving one or both ovaries with pelvic extension	III Peritoneal implants or positive lymph nodes	IV Distant metastasis, e.g. liver
5-year survival	90%	60%–70%	15%–35%	5%–15%

Primary care management

Ovarian cancer often presents with non-specific signs and symptoms. These, although non-specific and common amongst the general population, must always been taken seriously, especially in women over 50 years of age and with family history of ovarian or breast cancer (two or more cases diagnosed in first-degree relatives). In approximately 10% of cases there are no clinical symptoms or signs.

Ovarian cancer is often dubbed a silent killer; a systematic review estimated that the overall 5-year survival rate from ovarian cancer is around 30% with the majority of cancers being diagnosed at an advanced stage. The late presentation could be due to vague non-specific symptoms.[4] Diagnosis of ovarian cancer by a primary care physician can often be difficult. This reflects the relative rarity of the disease. A full-time GP with a list size of 2000 patients will see a new ovarian cancer only every 5 years or so. Contrast this with breast cancer where five times as many women are diagnosed. Furthermore, awareness of breast cancer symptoms is much higher as compared to ovarian cancer.

In my last 24 years of general practice with a list size of 3500, I have only seen one case of ovarian cancer. Evidence from case control studies has shown that symptoms that occur on a persistent basis (particularly more than 12 times per month) can have a sensitivity of 85% and a positive predictive value of 0.2% – meaning 1 in 500 women would have ovarian cancer.[5,6]

History

NICE guidance recommends further investigations if a woman experiences any of the following symptoms on an almost daily basis.

Obtain details of the following complaints – duration, onset and severity:

- persistent abdominal or pelvic pain
- abdominal distension
- persistent abdominal bloating (not the bloating feeling that comes and goes)
- abdominal mass/swelling
- urinary frequency/urgency[1]
- abnormal/postmenopausal bleeding
- loss of appetite
- unexplained weight loss[1]
- back pain
- extreme fatigue
- altered bowel habits;[1] any woman 50 years or over presenting with symptoms suggestive of irritable bowel syndrome must be taken seriously.

Obtain a thorough past obstetric and gynaecological history, identifying any potential risk factors for ovarian malignancy. Enquire about any family history of gynaecological or breast cancer.

Examination

- On general examination signs such as cachexia or excessive weight loss might be evident.
- Abdominal examination should aim in identifying any abdominal masses, signs of ascites and lymphadenopathy.
- Speculum examination and bimanual palpation should be undertaken, in order to visualise the cervix and detect any pelvic masses. Smaller adnexal masses are more difficult to ascertain and reports suggest that only 45% of adnexal masses are detected by pelvic examination.[7]

Differential diagnosis of ovarian cancer:
- uterine fibroids
- benign ovarian mass
- diverticular disease
- irritable bowel syndrome
- ascites due to other causes: cardiac or liver failure
- distended bladder.

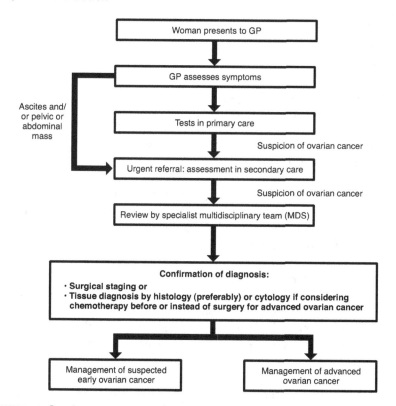

FIGURE 25.1 Ovarian cancer: overview of pathway

Investigations[1]

- Serum CA125 if a woman presents with symptoms suggestive of ovarian cancer.
- Patients with a CA125 of ≥35 IU should be referred for an ultrasound scan of the pelvis and abdomen including a TVUS. If both tests are abnormal, then the patient should be referred on the 2-week referral pathway. NICE recommends that these investigations should be requested by the GP prior to definitive referral. This obviously depends on GP access to these tests and the waiting time.
- If CA125 is within normal limits (<35 IU), NICE recommends careful assessment to exclude other clinical conditions.

CA125 is not highly sensitive nor specific and only 50% of stage 1 ovarian cancers have been found to have a raised CA125. If symptoms persist in spite of normal CA125, further investigations by referring the patient for pelvic ultrasound scan must be arranged.

Other causes of raised CA125:

- endometriosis
- pelvic infection
- fibroid
- ovulation.

A note on sonographic findings

When the pelvic ultrasound reports a suspicious ovarian mass, clearly a referral is indicated. In postmenopausal women, all ovarian cysts warrant referral to the gynaecological services as well as CA125 measurements.[1]

In premenopausal women, a simple cyst <50 mm can be managed by a repeat pelvic ultrasound in 3 months. If this disappears it means it was a functional cyst and no further follow-up is required. In case it persists referral is also indicated. For complex masses in premenopausal women, HCG, AFP and LDH should be obtained in addition to CA125, as there is a possibility of germ cell tumours.

Ovarian cancer screening

Screening using pelvic ultrasound, CA125 measurements or a combination of these has been studied. Common practice is to perform these two tests annually in women at high risk. It is generally agreed that at present, no strong evidence exists to support routine screening in any age group.

Management

Suspected ovarian cancer should be referred urgently to secondary care:[1]

- Women under the age of 40 years should have alpha-fetoprotein

(AFP), beta-human chorionic gonadotrophin (beta-HCG) and lactate dehydrogenase (LDH) checked to exclude germ cell tumours.

- A risk of malignancy index (RMI) should be calculated.

RMI combines three pre-surgical features: serum CA125, menopausal status (M) and ultrasound score (U).

RMI = U × M × CA125

The ultrasound score is scored 1 point for each of the: multilocular cysts, solid areas, metastasis, ascites and bilateral lesions.

U = 0 (for an ultrasound score of 0)

U = 1 (for an ultrasound score of 1)

U = 3 (for an ultrasound score of 2–5)

The menopausal score:

Premenopausal = 1

Postmenopausal = 3

Serum CA125 is measured in IU/mL and can vary between zero to hundreds or even thousands of units.

Refer to multidisciplinary team if RMI >250

- A CT scan of the abdomen and pelvis should be performed. CT of thorax should be carried out if clinically indicated.
- In tertiary centres an MRI scan of the pelvis is also carried out. This is not evidence-based and NICE does not recommend the routine use of MRI scan.
- Tissue diagnosis is a **must**.
- Every suspected cancer case must be discussed in a multidisciplinary gynae-oncology meeting, consisting of dedicated gynaecological oncologists. This decides whether treatment is required, the type of treatment and where it takes place (in district hospital/cancer unit versus in cancer centre).
- Patients with stage 1 must undergo optimal surgical staging. This consists of a midline laparotomy (to assess the pelvis and abdomen), peritoneal washings, total abdominal hysterectomy and bilateral salpingo-oophorectomy, infracolic omentectomy and removal of any macroscopic disease or suspicious lymph nodes.
- Patients with grade 3 or stage 1C are offered standard adjuvant chemotherapy, which normally consists of six cycles of carboplatin and

paclitaxel. Side effects include nausea, vomiting, alopecia, tiredness and neutropenia. Single agent carboplatin is used in patients with comorbidities.

- Chemotherapy for grade 2 stage 1A or 1B is debatable. The decision is made on the histological subtype.
- Patients with grade 1, stage 1A or 1B do not require adjuvant chemotherapy as recommended by NICE.
- For patients with stage 2–4, NICE recommends primary debulking surgery with adjuvant or neoadjuvant chemotherapy. NICE recommends a combination of paclitaxel with platinum-based compounds (carboplatin or cisplatin). If the patient is not fit for surgery, debulking is not recommended. The aim of debulking surgery is to resect all visible macroscopic disease.
- An ongoing trial supported by Cancer Research UK—Peritoneal Treatment of Ovarian Cancer (PETROC/OV21) is comparing three different types of chemotherapy for women who already had chemotherapy followed by surgery for ovarian cancer. In this study researchers are looking at giving different chemotherapy drugs given in different ways. The aim of the study is to find out if intraperitoneal chemotherapy helps women with ovarian cancer.[14]
- Prevention in BRCA-mutation carriers normally involves offering a risk reduction salpingo-oophorectomy at the age of 40 if a woman carries a BRCA1 mutation or 45 for a BRCA2 mutation. This can reduce the risk of ovarian cancer by up to 95%. This renders a woman menopausal and she may need HRT and testosterone replacement therapy.
- The combined contraceptive pill (COC) is of proven value for ovarian cancer prevention.[13] Use for 5 years or more reduces the risk by more than 50%.

Prognosis

Ovarian cancer is the leading cause of gynaecological cancer-related mortality, accounting for 6% of all cancer-related deaths.[8] The survival rate for women with ovarian cancer in the UK is significantly lower than the European average.[9] The 5-year survival rate has increased from 20% in 1975 to 38.9% in 2006. This could be due to early detection and early treatment and thus a better prognosis.[10]

- Ovarian cancer is the fifth most common cancer for women and the second most common gynaecological cancer.
- The three main symptoms common to most women are: abdominal distension that does not come and go; persistent pelvic or abdominal pain; and early satiety or loss of appetite.
- Diagnosis of ovarian cancer is often difficult because of the relative rarity of the cancer.
- If diagnosed in the early stages, survival rates can be as high as 90% but 3 out of 4 women are diagnosed once it has spread, decreasing survival rates dramatically.
- NICE recommends that serum CA125 should be the initial test followed by pelvic and abdominal ultrasound if the CA is ≥35 IU/mL.
- A normal CA125 does not exclude ovarian cancer.
- Women with suspected ovarian cancer should be referred on the 2-week cancer pathway to the local gynaecological cancer unit.
- Primary care has an important role in identifying and referring at-risk patients to the regional or local genetic services.
- Delayed or missed diagnoses of ovarian cancer and cancer of the cervix are the most common reason for medico-legal claims in general practice.[12]
- A CT scan of the abdomen and pelvis should be performed to establish the extent of disease.
- Women who have ovarian cancer should be managed by a cancer centre multidisciplinary team.[13]
- Surgery and chemotherapy – either individually or in combination – remain the therapeutic mainstay of treatment.
- For recurrent disease, chemotherapy is normally the treatment of choice.

Useful websites

For GPs

CancerStats key facts: ovarian cancer, Cancer Research UK: http://info.cancer researchuk.org/prod.consump/groups/cr_common/@nre/@sta/documents/general content/crukmig_1000ast-3058.pdf

Delayed diagnosis of cancer, National Patient Safety Agency: www.nrls.npsa.nhs.uk

Epithelial ovarian cancer, SIGN Publication No. 75: www.sign.ac.uk/pdf/sign75.pdf

NICE. Irritable bowel syndrome in adults: www.nice.org.uk/nicemedia/pdf/CG061NICEGuideline.pdf

NICE. Improving supportive and palliative care for adults with cancer: www.nice.org.uk/CSGSP

NICE. Guidance on the use of paclitaxel in the treatment of ovarian cancer: www.nice.
org.guidance/TA55

Ovarian Cancer Action: www.ovarian.org.uk/ovarian-cancer/

Management of Suspected Ovarian Masses in Premenopausal Women. Green-top
Guideline No 62. RCOG/BSGE Joint Guideline Nov 21. www.bogs.org.in/RCOG_
Guideline_Sukumar_Barik.pdf

Staging system for ovarian cancer, FIGO: www.targetovarian.org.uk/page.asp?section
=131&sectionTitle=FIGO+Stage+Classificatio+for+Ovarian+Cancer

For patients – helplines

Macmillan Cancerline: www.macmillan.org.uk

Ovacome ovarian cancer support network: www.ovacome.org.uk

Ovarian Cancer Action: www.ovarian.org.uk

Target Ovarian Cancer: www.targetovarian.org.uk

References

1 National Institute for Health and Clinical Excellence. Ovarian Cancer: the recognition and initial management of ovarian cancer: NICE guideline 122. London:
NIHCE; 2011. http://guidance.nice.org.uk/CG122

2 Target Ovarian Cancer. *FIGO Stage Classification for Ovarian Cancer.* www.
targetovariancancer.org.uk/page.asp?section=131...FIGO

3 Walsh P, Cooper N. Ovary. In: Quinn M, Wood H, Cooper N *et al. Cancer atlas
of the United Kingdom and Ireland 1991–2000.* Cardiff: Palgrave Macmillan; 2005.
pp 193–200.

4 Bankhead CR, Kehoe ST and Austoker J. Symptoms associated with diagnosis of
ovarian cancer: a systematic review. *BJOG.* 2005; 112: 857–65.

5 Hamilton W, Peters TJ, Bankhead C, *et al.* Risk of ovarian cancer in women with
symptoms in primary care population-based case-control study. *BMJ.* 2009; 339:
b2998.

6 Goff BA, Mandel LS, Drescher CW, *et al.* Development of an ovarian cancer symptom index: possibilities for earlier detection. *Cancer.* 2007; 109: 221–7.

7 Myers ER, Bastian LA, Havrilesky LJ, *et al.* Management of adnexal mass. *Evid
Rep Technol Assess.* 2006; 130: 1–145.

8 National Cancer Intelligence Network. *Cancer incidence and mortality by cancer
network, UK, 2005.* London: NCIN; 2008. Available at: www.ncin.org.uk/view.
aspx?rid=72 (accessed 16 December 2012).

9 Berrino F, Verdecchia A, Lutz JM, *et al.* The EUROCARE working group: comparative cancer survival information in Europe. *Europ J Cancer.* 2009; 45: 901–8.

10 Rachet B, Maringe C, Nur U, *et al.* Population-based cancer survival trends in
England and Wales up to 2007: an assessment of the NHS cancer plan for England.
Lancet Oncology. 2009; **10**(4): 351–69.

11 Hannaford PC, Iverson L, Macfarlane TV, *et al.* Mortality among contraceptive pill users. *BMJ.* 2010; 340: c927.

12 Esmail A, Neale G, Elstein M, *et al. Patient safety: lessons in litigation. Case studies in Litigation: Claims review in four specialities.* Manchester: Manchester Centre for Healthcare Management, University of Manchester; 2004. Available at: http://www1.imperial.ac.uk/resources/5DD55354-E618-416B-BC8F-9D599AEDA3AE/casestudyoflitigation.pdf

13 Department of Health. *Improving outcomes in gynaecological cancers.* London: Department of Health; 1999. Available at: www.dh.gov.uk/en/Publicationsand statistics/Publications/PublicationsPolicyAndGuidance/DH_4005385 (accessed 16 December 2012).

14 Cancer Research UK. *PETROC/OV21 – Peritoneal Treatment of Ovarian Cancer.* www.cancerresearchuk.org/science/research/who-and-what-we-fund/browse-by-location/london/university-college-london/grants/chris-gallagher-10994-cruk-09-015-petroc-ov21---peritoneal-treatment

26

Colposcopy

The introduction of an organised national screening programme in the UK in 1988 has been highly effective in terms of reducing mortality and morbidity. The incidence of cervical cancer fell by 42%.[1] Cervical cancer is the 11th most common cancer among women in the United Kingdom, accounting for around 2% of all new cases of cancer in females. In 2009, there were 3378 new cases of cervical cancers in the United Kingdom.[2] Cervical cancer is related to age but it does not follow the usual pattern of increase in incidence with increasing age. There are 2 peaks: the first in women aged 30–34 years and second in women aged 80–84 years.[2] The earlier peak is due to increased sexual activity giving rise to increase in human papillomavirus (HPV) – a precursor to cervical cancer. 76% of cervical cancers occur in the 25–64 years age group.

Mortality rates increase with age with the highest number of deaths occurring in the 75–79 age group. About 7 per cent of cervical cancer deaths occur in women under the age of 35 years.[3]

The latest relative survival figures for England show that around 67 per cent of women diagnosed with cervical cancer between 2005 and 2009 were alive five years later[3]

Risk Factors[3]

- Some types of HPV, in particular HPV 16 and HPV 18.[3] There is strong evidence that genital HPV infection is a cause of cervical cancer.[4] Genital HPV infection occurs almost exclusively as a result of sexual contact. The use of durex can effectively reduce the risk of male to female transmission.[5]
- Multiple sexual partners or where partners have had many sexual partners.
- Women taking immunosuppressive drugs after an organ transplant.

242

- HIV positive.
- Long term use of oral contraceptives but the benefit of taking oral contraceptives far outweigh the risks associated.
- Women who smoke are twice as likely to get cervical cancer.

TABLE 26.1 Timing of routine cervical smear invitation

AGE	FREQUENCY OF INVITATION
England, Northern Ireland and Wales	
25–49	3 yearly
50–64	5 yearly
Scotland	
20–60	3 yearly
From 2015	
25–49	3 yearly
50–64	5 yearly

The timings for cervical screening in England were changed in 2004. Women are now invited every 3 years from age 25–49 and every 5 years from age 50–64 years, with similar programmes in the rest of the UK. The changes arose as a result of a study by Cancer Research UK, which showed that while 3-year screening at 55–69 years offered a protection against invasive cancer of 87%, 5-year screening was almost as effective, offering protection of 83%. In the 40–54-year age group, the protection offered by yearly screening was 88% while 3-yearly screening was 84%. In younger women, screening is not as effective since the incidence is low, but progression from pre-cancerous changes to invasive cancer appears to be faster. The protection offered by 3-yearly screening in this age group is 61%, significantly greater than the 30% protection offered by 5-yearly screening.

Northern Ireland changed the ages and timings for cervical screening in line with England, with effect by January 2011.[11] Wales and Scotland followed in 2013; the changes in Wales to be implemented during 2013[12] and those in Scotland to be implemented in 2015.[13]

Invasive cervical cancer is rare in under 25s, the number of cases picked up by screening is very small and screening does not appear to be successful in detecting the cancers in this age group as compared to older age group.[6]

Cervical screening is designed primarily to identify not cancerous but potentially pre-cancerous changes. Women with many stages of abnormality are referred for colposcopy.[5] Treatments depend on findings at colposcopy but range from laser ablation or cold coagulation treatment, through laser excision or loop biopsy or hysterectomy for invasive cancer.

TABLE 26.2 Guidance for action on cervical smear results

GRADE	ACTION
Negative	Routine recall after 3 to 5 years
Abnormal	Refer for colposcopy after 3 abnormal tests at any grade in a 10-year period
Mild dyskaryosis	Ideally refer for colposcopy but it is acceptable to recommend a repeat test; if two tests are reported as mild dyskaryosis refer for colposcopy
Moderate dyskaryosis	Refer for colposcopy
Severe dyskaryosis	Refer for colposcopy
Suspected invasive cancer	Urgent 2-week referral
Inadequate	Repeat the test; refer for colposcopy after 3 consecutive inadequate samples

Colposcopy

A colposcopy is a detailed examination of the cervix (the neck of the womb) that allows the colposcopist (a specially trained doctor or nurse) to see the type and area of abnormality. This is performed using a magnifying instrument called a colposcope. Green light filters and solutions are used including acetic acid and iodine.

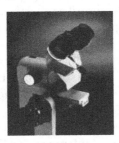

FIGURE 26.1 Colposcope

The colposcopy service:
- accepts referrals from path lab and GPs, and other colleagues
- diagnoses conditions from colposcopy examination
- takes samples from the cervix (a biopsy) to obtain a histological diagnosis
- treats the condition
- follows up treatment with further investigation if necessary
- discharges the patient back to the call-recall system

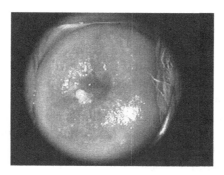

FIGURE 26.2 3% Acetic acid applied to cervix

- runs a failsafe system for checking the follow-up of all patients treated
- this service is provided in the gynaecology and some genitourinary medicine departments of the general hospital.

The majority of referrals to colposcopy are for women with abnormal cervical cytology results. These are made directly from the pathology lab to the colposcopy department. Direct referral to colposcopy following an abnormal smear result replaces the traditional referral route via primary care. It has been shown to improve service quality and reduce waiting times. Direct referral is in place for all grades of smear abnormality requiring colposcopy referral.

The HPV Sentinel Sites Implementation Project[7] has led to HPV triage of borderline changes and mild dyskaryosis, and testing has now been introduced into the cervical screening program. Where HPV triage is implemented, any woman who has a cervical screening test result of borderline changes or mild dyskaryosis will automatically have an HPV test performed on her sample. If HPV is found she will be referred for colposcopy and if HPV is not found she will be returned to routine screening every 3 or 5 years depending on her age.

Referral Guidelines for colposcopy: Cancer waiting times: North West Cervical Screening Quality Assurance Reference Centre (NWCSQARC 20 May 2010)[8]

- Where women are referred from the screening programme to colposcopy services they will be included within the 62 day standard introduced by the Cancer Reform Strategy. Women referred from primary care with moderate dyskaryosis or worse should be fast tracked as Urgent GP Referral for Suspected Cancer (Two-Week-Wait). This includes women with a cytology result of ?invasive or ?glandular if the local service protocol requires cytology result to be sent to patient's GP for action. In all such cases, a direct referral to colposcopy is strongly recommended. The receipt of this referral will be the starting point of both the 2-week period and the 62-day referral to treatment period. The receipt of this referral at the acute provider will also be the starting point for the 18 week commitment if cancer is later excluded by colposcopic examination or by biopsy.

- Patients diagnosed with cancer should receive their first definitive treatment within 31 days of agreeing their care plan or by 62nd day on their pathway whichever is sooner.
- All clinical procedures should be in the best interest of the patient and should not be influenced by the waiting time commitments. If a histological report is available, then this should be used to decide the future treatment pathway.
- Women with a cytology report of ?invasive cancer or ?glandular neoplasia should be seen within 2 weeks of referral.
- Women with a cytology report of moderate or severe dyskaryosis and who are on the 62-day pathway, should be seen in the colposcopy clinic within 4 weeks of referral.
- Women with a cytology report of borderline or mild dyskaryosis and who are on the 18-week pathway should be seen within 8 weeks of referral.
- Women with three consecutive inadequate samples should be referred for colposcopy.

Examination should be performed by a gynaecologist experienced in the management of cervical disease (such as a cancer lead gynaecologist).[9]

Other referral indications to colposcopy:
- Women presenting with post-coital bleeding (particularly women over the age of 40 years). Although post-coital bleeding is a cardinal sign of cervical neoplasia, the majority of cases are not malignant. In younger women, chlamydial infections are more likely causes. These women require appropriate assessment and referral for colposcopy if cancer is suspected.[8]
- Women with a history of intermenstrual bleeding.
- Blood stained vaginal discharge.

Treatment
Most treatment of abnormal cervical cells (if needed) can be carried out at colposcopy. Treatment depends on the full clinical picture of each individual patient, taking into account her age, parity and clinical findings.

Treatment options include the following.

Excisional treatments:
- large loop excision of the cervical transformation zone (LETZ)
- laser cone excision
- knife cone biopsy.

Destructive therapy:
- ball diathermy
- cold coagulation
- laser.

Post treatment, patients are followed up usually 6 months later with repeat cytology, HPV and test of cure. HPV 'test of cure' is being introduced for women who have undergone treatment for CIN. This means that HPV tests will be carried out on samples from women who have a normal, borderline or mild screening test result after treatment for CIN. If HPV is not found then a woman will not be recalled for screening for a further 3 years. If it is found, or the screening test does show an abnormality, the patient will be referred again to colposcopy.

Discharge from colposcopy

Colposcopy units are required to follow the North West Cervical Screening Quality Assurance Reference Centre (NWQARC) process at discharge.[8] This is to ensure that the local screening call/recall agency is notified when the patient is discharged from colposcopy. It is important that the local screening call/recall agency is notified when a patient is discharged so it can advise of a date for a follow-up smear, ensuring that the patient receives an invitation for that repeat smear at the appropriate interval.

Common appearances of the cervix

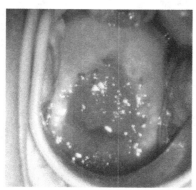

FIGURE 26.3 Normal ectopy

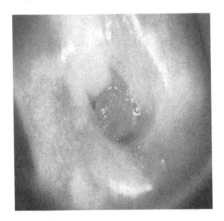

FIGURE 26.4 Cervical polyp

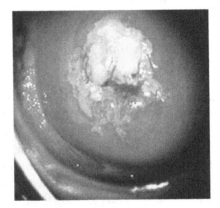

FIGURE 26.5 Acetowhite changes on colposcopy

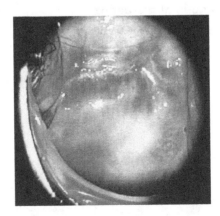

FIGURE 26.6 Totally stenosed os post-treatment

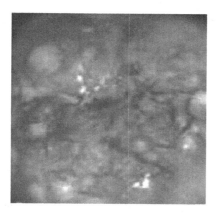

FIGURE 26.7 Nabothian follicles

Uncommon findings

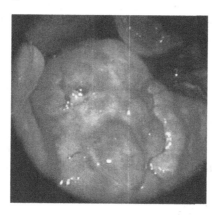

FIGURE 26.8 Small cell cancer of the cervix

KEY POINTS

- Cervical screening prevents most cases of cervical cancers.
- HPV is responsible for almost all cases of cervical cancer with types 16 and 18 accounting for majority of cases.
- Type 6 and 11 HPV account for about 90% cases of genital warts[9] and 10% cases of low grade CIN 1.[10]
- Multiple sexual partners, early age at first sexual intercourse and smoking are other possible risk factors.
- Gardasil, the quadrivalent vaccine,is licensed for the prevention of cervical cancer, CIN 2/3, genital warts and CIN 1 caused by types 6, 11, 16 and 18.

- Treatments depend on findings at colposcopy but range from laser ablation or cold coagulation treatment, through laser excision or loop biopsy to hysterectomy for invasive cancer.

References

1 NHS Cancer Screening Programmes. *Cervical screening: a pocket guide.* Available at: www.cancerscreening.nhs.uk/cervical/publications/cervicalpocket2004.pdf (accessed 16 December 2012).

2 Cancer Research UK. *Cervical cancer incidence statistics.* www.cancerresearchuk.org/cancer-info/cancerstats/types/cervix/incidence/uk-cervical-cancer-incidence-statistics (accessed Feb 2013).

3 NHS Cancer Screening Programmes. *Overview of cervical cancer in England – incidence, mortality and risk factors.* www.cancerscreening.nhs.uk/cervical/cervical-cancer.html (accessed February 2013).

4 Walboomers JM, Jacobs MV, Manos MM, *et al.* Human papillomavirus is a necessary cause of invasive cervical cancer worldwide. *J Pathol.* 1999; 189: 12–19.

5 Winer R, Hughes J, Feng Q, *et al.* Condom use and the risk of genital human papillomavirus infection in young women. *N Engl J Med.* 2006; 354: 2645–54.

6 Sasieni P, Adams J and Cuzick J. Benefit of cervical screening at different ages: evidence from the UK audit of screening histories. *Br J Cancer.* 2003; 89: 88–93.

7 NHS Cancer Screening Programmes. *HPV Sentinel Sites Implementation Project – NHS Cervical Screening Programme.* www.cancerscreening.nhs.uk/cervical/hpv-sentinel-sites-summary-sheet.pdf

8 NHS Cancer Screening Programmes. *Colposcopy and programme management: guidelines for the NHS Cervical Screening Programme.* 2nd ed. NHSCSP publication no. 20. Sheffield; 2010. Available at: www.cancerscreening.nhs.uk/cervical/publications/nhscsp20.pdf (accessed 27 March 2013).

9 von Krogh G. Management of anogenital warts (condylomata acuminata). *Eur J Dermatol* 2001; 11(6): 598–603.

10 Clifford GM, Rana RK, Franceschi S *et al.* Human papillomavirus genotype distribution in low grade cervical lesions: Comparison by geographic region and with cervical cancer. *Cancer Epidemiol Biomarker Prev.* 2005; 14(5):1157–64.

11 Northern Ireland Executive. *Cervical screening age to be raised in Northern Ireland.* Belfast; July 2010. Available at: www.northernireland.gov.uk/news/news-dhssps/news-dhssps-july-2010/news-dhssps-27072010-cervical-screening-age.htm (accessed 27 March 2013).

12 Llywodraeth Cymru Welsh Government. *Changes to cervical screening in Wales announced.* Cardiff; January 2013. Available at: http://wales.gov.uk/newsroom/healthandsocialcare/2013/130122cervicalscreeningagechange/?lang=en (accessed 27 March 2013).

13 Scottish Government Riaghaltas na h-Alba. *NHS Scotland: cervical screening.* Edinburgh; December 2012. Available at: www.scotland.gov.uk/News/Releases/2012/12/cervical-screening11122012 (accessed 27 March 2013).

Index

Entries in **bold** denote tables; entries in *italics* denote figures.

Printed in the United States
by Baker & Taylor Publisher Services